24·95

D0533895

MAKING SENS[
RISK MANAGEMENT

A workbook for primary care

Second Edition

In a nutshell . . . What you really need to know about risk management,
clinical governance and law and ethics

Roy Lilley and Paul Lambden

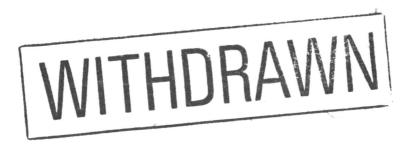

* 000209861 *

Radcliffe Publishing
Oxford • Seattle

Radcliffe Publishing Ltd
18 Marcham Road
Abingdon
Oxon OX14 1AA
United Kingdom

www.radcliffe-oxford.com
Electronic catalogue and worldwide online ordering facility.

© 2005 Roy Lilley and Paul Lambden

First edition 1999

British Library Cataloguing in Publication Data

A catalogue record for this book is available from the British Library.

ISBN 1 85775 713 0

Typeset by Anne Joshua & Associates, Oxford
Printed and bound by TJ International Ltd, Padstow, Cornwall

CONTENTS

PREFACE

It is five years since the first edition of this book. In that time a great deal has changed.

The concept of local Primary Care Groups coinciding with natural geographical boundaries and alignment with other local service providers seems to be a distant memory. PCGs have merged, disappeared and given way to PCTs, who have now become PCOs. Regional Health Authorities are a thing of the past, they are now 'strategic'. Foundation Trusts are the Government's flagship policy and as if to go full circle, it looks as though practice-based commissioning will reinvent something very like the GP fundholding policies of the early nineties.

The new General Medical Services Contract has emerged. Its birth seemed to be more the product of exasperation than careful thought about the future of primary care. Some say it marks the end of traditional vocational medicine.

Patients are starting to look back, fondly, to the times when they would go and see his or her 'own GP'. Like it or not, the practice of medicine and the practices themselves have changed forever.

Changed, too, is the environment in which medicine is practised. It is a litigious environment. An environment where risks must be identified in advance, hazards predicted and responses tailored and measured.

The media are full of stories about doctors' errors and health service foul-ups. The Government encourages the public to complain. TV and radio advertisements on behalf of solicitors prepared to work on a no-win, no-fee basis are endemic.

In the first edition of this book we said that there is no sin in getting something wrong. It could happen to a saint. The sin is failing to handle it properly when it does go wrong. It is important to recognise the problem, to act quickly to minimise the adverse consequences, to apologise where appropriate and to take steps to ensure that it doesn't go wrong again. Eliminating risk is what lets you sleep at night.

That was then and this is now. We stand by the advice and we wouldn't change it. Except that the sins have taken on the proportion of a felony!

Risk management is simple enough – work out what can go wrong and plan for the eventuality. An up-market version of Murphy's Law ('If something can go wrong it will'). The smart thing is to spot a problem in the making and do something about it in advance.

This is a 'do something about it' kind of book. Not rocket science, just common sense.

As we told you in 1999, you can decide to stay in bed and pull the covers over your head. On the other hand, if you need to earn a living, and you want it to be as stress-free as possible, try making sense of risk management.

We hope this book helps!

Paul Lambden
Roy Lilley
February 2005

ABOUT THE AUTHORS

Dr Paul Lambden BSc MB BS BDS FDSRCSEng MRCS(Eng) LRCP(Lond) DRCOG MHSM graduated in Medicine, Dentistry and Science at Guy's Hospital London. After working initially in Oral Surgery and obtaining his Fellowship of the Royal College of Surgeons of England, he entered general medical and general dental practice, continuing the two for over 15 years. He was also a clinical tutor at St Bartholomew's Hospital, London.

In 1992 he left general practice to become the Chief Executive of East Hertfordshire NHS Trust, a whole district trust providing services for 300 000 people with a budget of over £65 million. He was also appointed a specialist adviser to the all-party Parliamentary Health Select Committee, which he fulfilled for three years. In the late 1990s he became the Medical and Dental Principal of The St Paul International Insurance Company when it launched its professional indemnity (medical defence) programme for doctors and dentists.

More recently he has worked as managing director of MIA General Insurance and is currently working at Howden Medical Insurance Services. He was previously Lecturer in Law and Ethics at the Kigezi International School of Medicine at Cambridge.

Paul is a regular writer on healthcare, management and medical defence topics. He has made a number of programmes for medical television channels and has co-authored half a dozen textbooks with Roy Lilley including such subjects as the Internet, law and ethics, the Human Rights Act and risk management in medicine and dentistry.

Roy Lilley is a writer and broadcaster on health and social issues. He is the originator of the best-selling *Tool Kit* series of books on health service management and has written or co-written over 20 books. Formerly he was a visiting fellow at the Management School, Imperial College, London.

As a first-wave NHS Trust Chairman, his trust became the first in the UK to achieve BS 5750 (ISO 9001) quality accreditation for the whole of their services along with Investors in People approval for the whole of the HR and training strategies. Roy now works across the NHS to help with the challenges of modern management and is an enthusiast for radical policies that address the real needs of patients, professionals and the communities they serve.

DEDICATION

To our wives, who seem, intuitively,
to be better at managing risk than we are!

INTRODUCTION

OK, we know, you're not going to read this book from cover-to-cover.

Risk, law and ethics? Clinical Governance? What a bodice ripper!

Fear not! If you have a low boredom threshold, short attention span or lots of other interests, so do we! This is the book for you.

It is divided into short, distinct sections, each of which can be read in isolation. Only the anorak wearers are expected to read more than a few pages at a time. For the rest, look at it between patients, in the bath, on the loo or during the adverts on the telly.

Some of it will be of no interest to you. Skip past those bits. Pick out those parts that look as though they may actually be useful. Make sure that the kettle is on and that you have a nice biscuit to go with the regular cups of tea and coffee.

So, start as you mean to go on, make a brew and flick through the book.

Welcome back!

You will have noticed that law, ethics and risk management do not appear as separate sections. This is because they can be too boring and dense, so we've rolled them together, inter-relating them.

Smart readers will have spotted that the theories of ethics and the details of the law are also missing. They are left out on the 'you don't need to understand an engine to drive a car' principle.

Think boxes are there to get you thinking – obvious really. Some of them are provocative and some are there for a shameless bit of fun.

Hazard warnings – tricky issues or to avoid, career-threatening stuff, or things to keep you awake at nights.

☑

Tips are shortcuts and quick fixes that will get you to an answer faster, or they might just be good stuff worth taking special note of.

☺

Exercises are issues for you to work on and to use as ideas for brainstorming, for discussion with colleagues, or just to help you get your ideas straight – or a bright idea worth noting and taking some action on.

✍

Make a note – designed to remind you that something needs to be done, or borne in mind for the future.

Time to take a break and maybe reflect on something.

http://www . . . There are plenty of web addresses where you can find more detail. They come with a health warning. Web addresses are notorious for changing or disappearing altogether. At the time of going to press they were all nicely up-to-date. If, by the time you get there, they are not – sorry! Try Googling the topic and see if you can find some help. Also, some of the long web addresses may change. If you have a problem, try just the first part of the address and navigate your way to what you want from the opening page.

☺ This book is written, for the most part, in the second person. It seems friendlier that way.

However, some of the sections are clearly aimed at GPs and others – managers, receptionists, nurses, health visitors and admin staff.

In other words, the practice team. We don't see any reason why a manager shouldn't read the bits for the docs and the docs read the bits for the receptionist and so on. That way everyone gets a feel for the challenges, risks and problems facing each other.

And it's interesting isn't it?

Risk management (Roy's version!)

The term is made up of two words:

- **Risk** (n. & v.) – n. A chance or possibility of danger. Loss, injury or other adverse consequence.
- **Management** – n. The professional administration of business concerns.
- **Risk management** – Incomprehensible guru-speak and a task that is someone else's job.

Here's a proper definition (from Paul)!

- **Risk management** is a quality control related discipline comprising activities designed to minimise the adverse effects of loss upon a healthcare professional's physical, professional and financial assets by identifying any potential loss and reducing or preventing it.
- **Ethics** is the science of the morals of human conduct and provides the principles that rule the behaviour of society.
- **Law** is the enactment of custom or statute which is recognised as permitting or prohibiting certain actions and which is enforced by the imposition of penalties.

The strand that links ethics, law and risk is that primary care practices provide a standard expected by society, identified by ethics, upheld by law and with breaches minimised by risk management.

That's the explanations out of the way. Rip out the bits you like, dump the bits you don't and . . . good luck.

THE HIERARCHY OF RISK

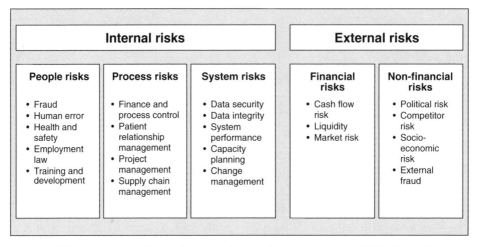

Internal risks			External risks	
People risks	**Process risks**	**System risks**	**Financial risks**	**Non-financial risks**
• Fraud • Human error • Health and safety • Employment law • Training and development	• Finance and process control • Patient relationship management • Project management • Supply chain management	• Data security • Data integrity • System performance • Capacity planning • Change management	• Cash flow risk • Liquidity • Market risk	• Political risk • Competitor risk • Socio-economic risk • External fraud

The sensible practice acknowledges that risks are a part of life, but the team does not take risks knowingly and tries to think about the things that can go wrong and takes steps to see that they don't. A sound system of internal controls helps to develop strategies, processes and contingency plans to prioritise the practice's efforts in favour of those events that are most likely to cause the most damage or lead to the greatest losses to the practice's investment, assets and reputation.

ORGANISATIONAL RISK MANAGEMENT

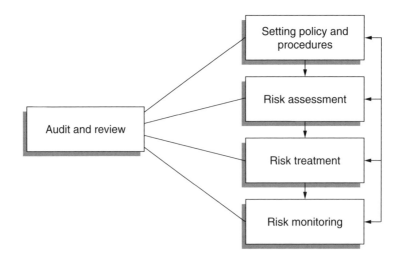

RISK MANAGEMENT

There is no doubt that, across the board, claims are increasing. The medical profession is no exception. Claims against doctors and practices are on the increase, too. Why? For five main reasons:

1 The public is more litigious and less tolerant of a medical outcome that is less than ideal.
2 It has become much more acceptable – perhaps even fashionable – to complain.
3 The Government encourages complaints about all public services.
4 There are increasing items in the media about poor healthcare.
5 There have been changes in the legal framework, particularly the advent of no-win, no-fee arrangements, that encourage claims.

Practices do not have to give up and think a claim is inevitable. By applying some simple risk management principles, the likelihood of a complaint or a claim can be markedly reduced.

Risk management in guru-speak:

> '. . . is a quality control related discipline comprising activities designed to minimise the adverse effects of loss upon a health-care professional's physical, professional and financial assets by identifying any potential loss and reducing or preventing it.'

Here are the four simple Principles of Risk Management, in plain English:

1 **Identify the risk:** What can go wrong?
2 **Analyse the risk:** How likely is it to go wrong and how serious an impact might it have?

☺ **Exercise**

Let's start with the basics and the blindingly obvious. Have a look at the practice and see what risks you are exposed to – the dodgy electric plug, the dangling wire, the curly edge of a carpet. It takes 10 minutes and may save a fortune in claims!

---

3 **Control the risk:** What can you do to reduce or eliminate it or transfer it to someone else?
4 **Cost the risk:** What is the cost of getting it right versus the cost of getting it wrong?

Remember, a claim from a damaged patient not only has financial and professional consequences but often severe personal and emotional consequences as well.

Increased exposure to risk may occur for a variety of reasons.

- Not being up to date with the latest best practice, guidance or technology.
- Managing a situation badly and a complication develops with a patient's care.
- A failure of continuity of care.
- A breakdown in communication.
- Failure to act to maintain the practice's assets.
- Failure to properly manage finance.
- Actions that lead to damage to reputation.
- Actions that lead to damage to relationships with family, colleagues or staff.

>  **Tip**
>
> It is everyone's job to be aware of risk management. Encourage it, support it, reward it and be pleased when staff spot a problem. Don't shout at them for whingeing!

It is everyone's job to reduce or eliminate the risks associated with practice. Only by doing so will claims be kept under control and huge rises in insurance premiums be minimised.

In some occupations a bad claims history already causes difficulty for the affected professional in obtaining indemnity. And without insurance you cannot work!

> ☑ **Tip**
>
> Try the Post-It Note Challenge. Give some post-it notes to everyone in the practice, ask them to go round the building making a note and sticking a post-it note on everything that appears hazardous. You might be surprised by the result!

THE DUTIES OF A GENERAL PRACTITIONER

All the mainstream orthodox medical professions have regulatory bodies and clear-cut codes of practice and standards. The codes for the six principal healthcare professions – doctors, dentists, nurses, osteopaths, chiropractors and physiotherapists – are remarkably similar and confer similar, onerous professional burdens on practitioners.

> Promoting Excellence? Does that have any regard for resources?

The regulatory body for GPs is the General Medical Council (GMC) and it fulfils a number of functions:

- It protects patients by promoting excellence in medical care.
- It regulates, develops and promotes the profession by:
  - maintaining a register of those doctors who are appropriately qualified and can demonstrate safe practice of the profession
  - defining standards of education, training and clinical practice
  - dealing promptly with doctors whose competence or fitness to practise is called into question
  - developing the profession and the practice of medicine.

The GMC has been overseeing and regulating the medical profession since it was established under the Medical Act of 1858. It has strong and effective legal powers designed to maintain the standards that the public have come to expect. The GMC has produced a set of criteria, compliance with which should ensure that the profession maintains a good standard of practice and shows appropriate respect for human life.

☺ Of course, all doctors read these criteria every day but, just in case you haven't had your fix today, these are your duties. As a doctor you must:

- make the care of your patient your first concern
- treat every patient politely and considerately
- respect patients' dignity and privacy
- listen to patients and respect their views
- give patients information in a way they can understand
- respect the rights of patients to be fully involved in decisions about their care
- keep your professional knowledge and skills up to date
- recognise the limits of your professional competence
- be honest and trustworthy
- respect and protect confidential information
- make sure that your personal beliefs do not prejudice your patients' care
- act quickly to protect patients from risk if you have good reason to believe that you or a colleague may not be fit to practise
- avoid abusing your position as a doctor; and
- work with colleagues in the ways that best serve patients' interests.

In all these matters you must never discriminate unfairly against your patients or colleagues. And you must always be prepared to justify your actions to them.

After all this a cup of coffee is in order!

Is complying with this code demanding? True, it requires actions and behaviour of the highest standards, yet the profession would not be able to act without standards. Patients must feel they can trust GPs. They must feel sure that they understand what will happen to them and that information they provide will be kept secure.

As skills evolve, all professionals must keep up to date and compliments and complaints should both receive prompt responses.

Finally, the GP must be prepared to notify the GMC if he or she becomes aware of a practitioner who may damage patients or whose behaviour brings the profession into disrepute. Failure to meet this latter standard may have serious consequences for a GP. If a patient suffers harm as a result of a practitioner's incompetence or ill-health and the deficiency is known to another GP and that knowledge subsequently comes to light, the GP may find him or herself brought before the GMC to explain and justify why he or she did not make the report. The punishment for failure of the doctor to report could be as severe as that for the doctor whose performance was compromised.

It is the code of practice that holds the profession in good stead with society and which elevates the practitioners above those healthcare professions in the more peripheral specialities where questions of quality and standard remain unresolved because no such codes exist.

☺ **Exercise**

Which of the following incidents or circumstances should you notify to the insurer?

- a patient who develops haematuria after you have injected his piles
- someone who feels that you have breached confidentiality to his wife
- someone who claims that you have undertaken treatment for which she did not consent
- a patient who had symptoms suggestive of a spinal tumour but who you forgot to refer to a specialist for two weeks.

ANSWER: All of them, of course. If anything at all happens, let the insurance company know.

PROFESSIONAL INDEMNITY REQUIREMENTS

In recent years GPs have seen some dramatic changes in their indemnity arrangements. Costs of premiums have risen rapidly as the number of claims and their associated legal costs have increased. Traditionally, professional indemnity has been provided by three defence organisations: the Medical Protection Society, the Medical and Dental Defence Union of Scotland and the Medical Defence Union. All three organisations have been in existence for over a century. More recently The St Paul International Insurance Company entered the market in 1999, only to leave three years later after the events of September 11 2001. Recently another insurer has launched a new policy.

Here's the lowdown.

Indemnity may be provided within the insurance industry either on a **claims-made** or an **occurrence** basis. Claims-made cover is provided currently by the **Medical Defence Union** along with other insurers.

It does 'what it says on the tin'. With a **claims-made** arrangement, the policy

> How does the defence market operate? Is there likely to be a proliferation of defence organisations? Are they necessary?

responds to a **claim**. The term 'claim' is really a poor term because it implies that the insurer is only interested in situations where a GP receives a solicitor's letter alleging professional misconduct or where the General Medical Council notifies the GP of a complaint.

Not true! The insurer's interest is in fact much wider. It is a requirement to notify the company, not only about the big events mentioned above but also about patient complaints made verbally or in writing to the GP, about enquiries from patients or legal firms for copies or sight of the medical records (using the Data Protection Act 1998) and of **any incident or circumstance that might, later, give rise to any sort of claim.**

By contrast an **occurrence-based** cover provides indemnity depending on when the 'incident' occurred. The Medical Protection Society and the Medical and Dental Defence Union of Scotland both provide indemnity on this basis. The event in question may have taken place months or years earlier but as long as the indemnity was in place at the time of the incident the GP can seek assistance. An **occurrence** indemnifier needs to be notified of all the same events and incidents.

Got any questions so far? Of course you have:

IS A CLAIMS-MADE OR AN OCCURRENCE POLICY BETTER?

In reality, both types of indemnity meet the requirements of the practitioners to respond to claims provided the appropriate arrangements are in place.

However, there is a key difference. A **claims-made** policy responds to a 'claim'. At the end of any policy year the insurer will have received notification of a number of claims as a result of allegations against GPs. All the claims will either have been resolved (successfully defended or settled) or 'reserved' and an estimate made of the likely final costs involved in handling the claim.

The indemnifier will therefore have a good understanding of the total financial liability to which it will be exposed and can allocate funds to meet the claims accordingly. It is also able to ensure the appropriate setting of premium for the following year.

Because an occurrence indemnifier provides cover for incidents, the claim associated with any incident may arise weeks, months or years later. It is possible that a claim could arise 10, 20 or more years after the event. This can make reserve forecasting (putting aside sufficient money to meet claims that may arise in future) very difficult for a defence organisation because, at the end of a year of cover, it will have no idea whether it will receive further claims in the future and, if so, what their value will be.

WHAT IS THE DIFFERENCE BETWEEN DISCRETIONARY AND CONTRACTUAL COVER?

Potentially the issue of discretionary versus contractual cover is far more important. It depends on whether a doctor is indemnified by an insurance company or a mutual society. At present the current providers are as follows:

- mutual societies:
  - The Medical Protection Society
  - The Medical and Dental Defence Union of Scotland
- mixed insurer with a mutual society overlay:
  - The Medical Defence Union.

If any new indemnity (defence) organisations enter the market they will almost certainly be insurance companies and it is extremely unlikely that a new mutual society will appear.

Mutual societies originated as organisations where groups of individuals united to pool resources to defend themselves on a 'one for all, all for one' basis. Undoubtedly this was successful during the twentieth century but there is little doubt that increasing claims rates and rising legal costs may have placed some mutual societies under pressure. This is a worldwide phenomenon.

In 2002, United, the largest Australian mutual society, went into provisional liquidation when its reserves were inadequate to meet actual and anticipated claims. As a result the Australian Government changed the legislation to outlaw mutual medical defence organisations and to ensure that all cover provided was by insurance companies.

In the UK defence industry mutual societies have key differences from insurers:

- The cover they provide is **discretionary**. This means that the member has **no automatic right** to assistance or support if a claim is made against him or her but depends on the approval generally of the Council of the organisation. Clearly this is no problem when reserves are plentiful but if the organisation is under financial pressure, of the type experienced by United in Australia, many people fear that the practitioner may find him or herself exposed to huge financial liabilities. As a mutual society gives no automatic right to indemnity, it should more correctly be described as providing professional negligence services.

- There is no contract indicating what indemnity is actually provided because nothing is guaranteed and what is provided for one member may not be provided for another member seeking the same help.
- Mutual societies are not regulated by the Financial Services Authority. Indeed, because they are mutual discretionary organisations that can elect not to meet claims, there is no requirement for them to have reserves at set levels nor any requirement to demonstrate that they have sufficient funds to meet all claims.

Insurance companies operate on a fundamentally different basis:

- There is a **contract of insurance** that makes explicit to the policyholder what is and is not covered. This is sometimes criticised for building in exclusions whereas mutual societies cover 'everything'. The reality of the situation is that mutual societies contract to cover nothing at all.
- There is no discretion to reject any claim covered by the policy terms.
- The insurance companies are monitored by the Financial Services Authority and must comply with stringent financial requirements. They must be able to demonstrate that they have the funds to meet all known or potential claims.

And then there is 'run-off'

You need to know this!

Run-off is cover provided by a claims-made insurer to meet claims that may arise in the future after the active policy has been terminated.

If a policyholder ceases to have insurance, there could be a risk that a claim could be made for which he or she did not have cover, unless appropriate arrangements had been made. There has, on occasion, been a problem with GPs leaving a claims-made insurer.

In that situation some GPs have been asked to pay an additional charge to cover that eventuality. However, this would be unnecessary for GPs moving to another claims-made insurer if that insurer provides retrospective cover. Because a claims-made policy looks at when the **claim** is made, the incident may have occurred before the GP was insured. Provided the GP was unaware of any potential claim at the time he or she took out the insurance, the policy provides retrospective cover. The policy will respond to any appropriate claim. This is subject to the terms of the policy, as long as it occurs during the period of insurance. An occurrence policy only operates provided it was in force when the incident occurred.

How is a 'claim' managed?

The indemnifier will provide assistance and support when any incidents or circumstances are notified. Normally the first contact will be with a medico-legal adviser who will provide initial advice and, where a claim is identified, will work with the claims team, either in the mutual society or in the insurance company that underwrites the cover to ensure that the GP receives all necessary advice to react quickly. The GP should be informed and involved at all stages of the claims process.

Any high-quality medical defence organisation will have as its aim the provision of high-quality, rapid assistance to its members or policyholders.

All good defence organisations understand how distressing a claim may be and how important it is to be able to speak to another healthcare professional whenever it is necessary.

A GP's whole future could depend on it!

> If you have any concerns or problems associated with your professional activities, be sure your cover meets your requirements. You should be asking yourself whether the organisation has adequate reserves, whether it provides good medico-legal advice and whether it will be there to respond without question when you need it.

OK, take a break – enough complicated stuff. Time for another cuppa.

HANDLING COMPLAINTS

Complaints are on the increase across the whole spectrum of healthcare. Most complaints received by GPs are dealt with within the practice.

Every practice should have a nominated complaints manager, usually the practice manager, and he or she should be skilled, trained and really good at handling problems.

> 10 top tips for complaint handling
> 1 Keep the insurer informed.
> 2 Do not ignore complaints.
> 3 Act quickly and speak to the patient.
> 4 Do not write aggressive responses.
> 5 Do not omit the difficult bits.
> 6 A conciliator may help.
> 7 Do not get cross.
> 8 Don't go to an independent review alone.
> 9 The Ombudsman is independent.
> 10 It may be OK to say sorry.

Only a relatively small number of complaints go on to become claims or are lodged with the General Medical Council.

Receipt of a complaint is an important event. It must be handled effectively. Some authorities say that complaints are good and should be treated as a learning exercise. Others think they are a nuisance to be dealt with as quickly as possible. Whatever the viewpoint, a dissatisfied complainant can cause a lot of trouble for a GP.

Best practice suggests that the following principles should always be adopted:

1 **Keep your medical defence insurer informed:** The defence

> ✍ **Make a note**
> Insurers are set up to help with complaints. Let them know straight away if you get one. They understand that even the best GP can get a complaint and it is not seen as an automatic black mark. However, hiding a complaint may be seen as original sin.

organisation medico-legal advisers are used to dealing with complaints. It is often the case that the person to whom the complaint has been directed is the last person to respond in a calm and rational manner. You should telephone the advice line to find out the best course of action. You should receive advice on the reply and a review of your draft response letter to make sure that it uses appropriate wording. If you don't, change your insurer!

2 **Do not ignore complaints:** A complaint does not go away. Do not put it in a drawer and hope that you will not hear any more. You will, and next time it will be more aggressive and difficult to deal with.

3 **Act quickly and speak to the patient:** The evidence is that a speedy response is much more likely to resolve a problem than a slow one peppered with delays.

Although speaking to the patient is not ideal in every case, it is held that in most cases speaking to a dissatisfied patient can contribute to resolving the problem.

> **✎ Make a note**
>
> Healthcare professionals are expert at talking to patients, especially when the patients are cross or upset. Unless there is a good reason **not** to talk to someone, it is well worth the effort.
>
> If you do, do so in a relaxed atmosphere, offer them a cup of tea, have someone present (a receptionist or practice manager) taking notes (and who will give a copy of the notes to both you and the patient afterwards) and talk through the problem.
>
> Talk through this strategy with the insurer beforehand.

Talking to people – communicating – is what all healthcare professionals do and you should be very good at it. It is also important not to forget that complainants may have some justification and you never know, you might even learn something. However time-consuming meeting with a patient might be, it will probably be a lot quicker than the hours spent otherwise dealing with a protracted dispute.

4 **Do not write aggressive responses:** Telling a patient what you think of them in a complaint response may make you feel better, but it will be short-lived. The patient is very likely to write again, this time more aggressively, and will also be more prepared to complain to others, such as the GMC.

If you are going to respond aggressively you must be sure that you are absolutely right and that you have no regard for any consequences.

Consequences? Here's a few: regulatory body interest, bad publicity and damage to reputation. Enough? Get the picture?

Take into account not only to whom the letter is written but also who else may see it. Although it may be addressed to an individual who has complained, the likelihood is that it will be shown to others; friends, relatives, Citizens' Advice Bureau, etc. The complainant may even agree (at least privately) with what you have said but it may not sound so good to others who were less personally involved.

5 **Do not miss out difficult bits:** It is often the case that a complaint letter raises a number of issues. Even if one or more of the matters is embarrassing or difficult, it is unwise to leave it out in the hope that detailed answers to more minor complaints will distract the patient from the key issue. It will not. You will simply receive a further letter specifically directed to the difficult complaint, which will then be more awkward to answer effectively.

6 **A conciliator:** Sometimes complaints are complex

> ☺ **Light relief**
>
> Handling complaints is an art. Patient complaints are often colourful: here are a few that caused some consternation:
>
> - The GP's suggestion that the diagnosis would only be made at post mortem was entirely unacceptable.
> - When I tried to make an appointment, I discovered you were on holiday. The receptionist refused to give me your holiday address.
> - To be told that people as old and fat as me should not go to the gym was abrupt to the point of offence.

> ☺ **Oh dear**
>
> Sadly, replies in draft responses are often no better:
>
> - I am well-known for my obtuse manner.
> - I am naturally disappointed that my manipulation of your lumbar spine was ineffective but pleased that your appendicectomy was successful.
> - If I ever see you again it will be much too soon!

or have many facets and they may become bogged down in a morass of correspondence which may become acrimonious. In such circumstances a conciliator may be very helpful. Available through the PCT, the conciliator will seek agreement from both parties to be involved. He or she will then visit the complainant and establish the fundamental issues, visit the GP and explain the patient's concerns and seek answers from the practitioner and then return to see the patient, give the information and try to achieve a resolution. This is often successful in complaints that seem inexorable.

7 **Don't get cross:** This is really the ultimate sign of failure. If you lose your temper everything will break down and the complainant may well pass the issue on to someone else. That 'someone else' may be the GMC or a really ugly lawyer.

> ☺ Oh, go on, get cross. Write something really rude here!

8 **Do not go to an independent review on your own:** If a patient successfully applies for an independent review of the complaint, you should not attend on your own.

Take someone from your LMC, from your defence insurer, or a senior colleague.

Your 'friend' (who incidentally cannot be a solicitor) can watch out for your interests whilst you answer questions and can make sure that some amateur Perry Mason doesn't try to trick you into remarks that might have adverse consequences later.

9 **The Ombudsman may be a valuable resource:** If a doctor feels that he or she is badly treated by an independent review an application can be made to the Ombudsman to review the case. The Ombudsman is not there just for the patient. There have been cases where PCTs (and before them Health Authorities) have been obliged to apologise to GPs for the way in which hearings were conducted.

10 **It's OK to say sorry:** Listening to a complaint, sympathising and saying sorry is a simple and very effective way of diffusing criticism. 'I'm sorry you've had the pain', or 'I'm sorry you had to go through all that', is simple and sincere. You don't have to say you are an idiot and got it all wrong. It can be that your chosen course turns out to be wrong. If you've

done your honest best, it is not the end of your professional world. If your decisions are reviewed by other GPs and they agree you've done your best and acted appropriately, just as they might have done, then your world will keep turning.

What you must do is to use your professional skills to make a reasonable assessment of the patient and to provide the standard of care an ordinarily skilled GP would have provided. No one comes to work, intent on getting it wrong, but in the course of a GP's professional life, as with any other profession, something will go wrong. It is the measure of the person how they respond.

If you get a complaint tell your defence organisation immediately. Get help to manage the complaint and write the reply. If you can satisfy the patient and resolve the complaint quickly you will have a less stressful practising life and a much lower risk of a claim.

☑ After all, you don't want to meet an ugly lawyer, do you?

THE GENERAL MEDICAL COUNCIL
(or whatever comes next – *see* Annex)

The General Medical Council (GMC) is the regulatory body for all GPs. All GPs must be registered with the GMC to be able to practise and for the privilege of registration they must pay an annual retention fee.

The medical profession, like a number of other mainstream healthcare professions, enjoys self-regulation. In other words, the regulation of the profession (education, standards, keeping a register and discipline) is done by the profession itself rather than by an outside agency.

Following the *Shipman* case, the GMC has come under huge scrutiny and as a result, the Government has created statutory bodies such as the Council for Healthcare Regulatory Excellence (formerly known as the Council for the Regulation of Healthcare Professionals), which has powers to intervene in the disciplinary process (and which has done so in a few cases).

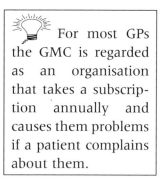 For most GPs the GMC is regarded as an organisation that takes a subscription annually and causes them problems if a patient complains about them.

In general their involvement to date has been in those cases where it was held that the GMC had been too lenient in cases where a doctor had been found guilty of professional misconduct.

From an insurance point of view, it is important not to incur the interest of the GMC if at all possible because hearings are traumatic for the GP and expensive for the insurer (with consequent implications for future premiums).

☑   If you are an insomniac, or an anorak, or have a problem lurking in the wings – here is everything you need to know about the GMC and complaints:

> 'The GMC was established in 1858, initially to distinguish between qualified and unqualified medical practitioners.'

The GMC's role subsequently expanded to include a variety of responsibilities including registration, education and disciplinary matters. In 2002 the Privy Council agreed legislation to introduce new GMC arrangements in three broad areas:

- Constitutional reform to reduce the governing body from 104 to 35 and increase lay membership from 24% to 40%. The first new Council took office in July 2003.
- Reform of fitness to practise procedures.
- Reform of the registration procedures including the introduction of revalidation to demonstrate that doctors meet the standards necessary for continued registration.

> ☺ Doctors will, in future, have a licence to practise. Just like a betting shop!

The powers of the GMC are set out in the Medical Act of 1983. It has been amended in subsequent years by a variety of other legislation.

The Council regulates and monitors GPs' fitness to practise. It is an integral part of the Council's duties to regulate the profession and protect the public and the profession's reputation.

The GMC has legal powers to act against doctors where it is alleged that a doctor has been guilty of professional misconduct or incompetence, convicted of a criminal offence or is impaired by health problems. Under the old system a decision was taken at an early stage to direct a complaint into one of three procedures: health, performance or conduct. Each potentially could have a different outcome and not all could result in the doctor being struck off the medical register. Cases were heard by members of the Council of the GMC.

Under the recently introduced new system, there is a new single complaints process. All complaints will go through the same process irrespective of their nature. The GMC's view is that this will enable the doctor's fitness to practise to be considered without being labelled early on as either a health, performance or conduct issue. The same outcomes and sanctions will be available to apply to every case, regardless of their type.

The panels that decide a case involving a doctor will have no GMC Council members sitting on them.

According to the GMC the new system will streamline the current processes, ensure that complaints progress promptly and are fair.

The number of complaints about doctors are remarkably few given the number of registered doctors in the United Kingdom. Data from the GMC itself shows the number of enquiries and complaints about doctors between 2001 and 2003 as follows:

Year	Number of complaints/enquiries
2001	4,504
2002	3,937
2003	3,962

In 2003 the following sanctions were imposed against doctors:

Erasures from the Register

At PCC	47
Voluntary	85
Others	10
Total erasures	**142**

Suspensions

Conduct/Conviction	20
Health	53
Performance	10
Total suspensions	**83**

Conditions imposed

Conduct/Conviction	31
Health	70
Performance	29
Total conditions	**130**

The GMC has an in-house legal team with up to 15 lawyers! Looks like they expect to be busy! Their purpose is to represent the GMC and to give advice to those people involved in case decision-making at every stage.

THE NEW COMPLAINTS PROCEDURE

The Council for Healthcare Regulatory Excellence (CHRE)

The CHRE is seen by many as a threat to the self-regulation of the nine statutory healthcare regulators in the United Kingdom.

It was established in April 2003 as the Council for the Regulation of Healthcare Professionals (CRHP) and its remit is fourfold:

> **Thought for the day**
>
> Spare a thought for the GMC. These days they find themselves in something of a dilemma. If they are too tough on GPs they end up being criticised by the profession but if they are too lenient, the Council for Healthcare Regulatory Excellence (CHRE) has the power to review the case and if they feel the GMC has not issued a suitable punishment, take it to the High Court.

- to promote the interests of the public and patients in relation to regulation of the healthcare professions
- to promote best practice in the regulation of the healthcare professions
- to develop principles for good professionally-led regulation
- to promote co-operation between regulatory bodies and other organisations.

The CHRE is an overarching, independent body that overseas the regulatory work of the nine regulating bodies, which are:

- the General Medical Council
- General Dental Council
- General Osteopathic Council
- General Chiropractic Council
- General Optical Council
- The Health Professions Council
- The Nursing and Midwifery Council
- The Royal Pharmaceutical Society of Great Britain . . .
- and the Pharmaceutical Society of Northern Ireland.

It is accountable to the Westminster Parliament and independent of the UK Departments of Health.

The significance for practitioners is that it has the power to appeal decisions of the regulatory bodies.

For example, if a decision by the GMC, finding a practitioner not guilty of serious professional misconduct, is judged in their gobbledy speak, as a 'relevant decision' it can be referred to court by CHRE under Section 29(4) of the National Health Service Reform and Health Care Professions Act 2002.

This effectively means that the CHRE can challenge 'not guilty' findings as well as unduly lenient sanctions.

Finally, the significance of the name change from the CRHP to the CHRE should be noted. From August 2004 it was no longer about regulating healthcare professionals, but it adopted a new role as the Council for Healthcare Regulatory Excellence.

Is this fair? A practitioner in this situation will, in effect, be exposed to a double jeopardy effect, having to defend him or herself in a regulatory body hearing, only to be subject to the possibility of referral and review of the whole case again by the High Court if found to be innocent or only guilty of a more minor offence.	☺ For doctors, particularly those subjected to scrutiny by the Council, after allegedly being 'treated too leniently' by the GMC, what difference will the name change make?

COMPETENCE AND CONTINUING PROFESSIONAL DEVELOPMENT

There's a lot of it about! Everybody is doing it.

What is it? Well, there is a book to be written on the definitions alone! All the professions and all the management organisations are getting into continuing professional development (CDP), in a big way. The truth is: they have to, and fortunately, it is a nice little earner for them.

If people are obliged to hone up their skills and keep up to date, it's a jolly good idea to sell them a personal development course, or two, to help them do it. So, when it comes to a definition, there's plenty of choice.

> ☺ In other words, bone up, hone up, keep up to date and up to scratch . . .

Here are the bare bones:

> '. . . a process that enables staff to acquire, maintain and enhance their knowledge, skills and attitude to optimise individual and organisational performance . . .'

Great emphasis is being placed on the significance and importance of CPD. The Gods of Whitehall also think it is very important to keep the workforce up to scratch. It makes for a safer environment for patients and a more efficient working environment.

Let's start with the basics.

KEEP A NOTE

It is vitally important to keep a written record of CPD activities – it's called a portfolio. That way you have a record to prove that you have been doing all the right things to develop your illustrious career and keeping up to date with all the new-fangled things that make life more complicated.

There is a little matter of 'accountability for performance', which means, in plain English, 'what you do is down to you'. Keeping a record of your CPD activities goes a long way in any argument about accountability.

GPs must keep a 'portfolio' of their CPD stuff. The RCGP www.rcgp.org.uk provides useful models, templates and guidance on what to do, as do most of the professional organisations for clinicians and managers.

WHAT DO YOU NEED TO KNOW?

This bit is called 'assessing your learning needs'. Not as easy as it seems. For example; how do you find out what you need to know, if you don't know what you need to know?

The trick is a useful little process called reflective practice.

> ☢ How do you find out what you need to know, if you don't know what you need to know?

WHAT ARE OTHER PEOPLE DOING?

Find out what leading-edge practitioners, managers and services are doing and do the same! This is all about being what management gurus call 'research-aware'. In other words, keeping your eyes

> ☑ As a professional, have you contacted another professional in a primary care organisation in the last week? If not why not?

open to what is going on and having a good old gossip (networking) whenever you can.

One of the best sources is learning from a peer group – other professionals in your line of business.

LEARNING WITH OTHERS

The Department of Health are very keen on the idea of teams. They keep on banging on about team-based learning. There is no doubt that modern service delivery, not just in

> ☺ Somewhere in your organisation is a good idea and a back that needs patting. Can you find them?

primary care, but everywhere in the public services, is a team-based business. Each is dependent on the skills and talents of the other. Team-based get-togethers, brainstorming and learning makes a lot of sense.

 . . . reflective practice?

   This needs the assistance of a cup of caffeine or something more relaxing and stronger. We guess it depends on the time of day!

   Think of a circumstance in your recent work that just didn't feel right. Perhaps a colleague raised a topic that you didn't know too much about. Perhaps you were at a meeting and didn't feel able to chip in and have your say?

   If it was uncomfortable, the chances are you didn't know about something that everyone else did.

> ☺ Don't forget, you can learn from success as well as failure. The things that make you feel good are just as worth reflecting on. They are usually the areas where you can really move forward in your learning and skills base.

Perhaps someone had a success, where you once didn't.

   Whatever it is that makes you reflect is usually a good place to start some learning.

RISK ASSESSMENT: WELL THIS IS WHAT THE BOOK IS ALL ABOUT!

Later in the book there is a section on clinical governance. Risk assessment and risk management is at the heart of clinical governance. It is also true of CPD. What you don't know is the really risky bit! Think about the things you do and the activities you undertake. How can they go wrong? What needs to be done to stop you and the practice from making errors? Answer the question and you will find yourself in the right place to think about your, and the organisation's, development needs.

THERE'S NEVER ENOUGH TIME

Time is precious. You can't make time or steal time, but you can organise time and invest time. 'Time' is no reason not to sort out CPD and it is no excuse. The point of the clinical governance agenda, which is tied to CPD, is that it is an organisational framework and an organisational responsibility.

Staff must have the opportunity to negotiate their objectives within an organisation and ensure that effective CPD is one of those objectives.

CPD needs access to information and these days that means information technology, computers and the Internet. How many practice staff have a desk to call their own and how many have the luxury of being able to sit in a library? Make sure there is Internet access for staff to sort out their learning needs.

PERSONAL DEVELOPMENT PLANS (PDPS)

The majority of health professional staff should have had PDPs in place by April 2000 (HSC 1999/154). Plans are not made in isolation. Although they are 'personal', they must meet the needs of the local population, as well as the personal and professional needs of the individual.

They have to be woven into the needs of the PCG.

The best way to check this is the case, is through an effective appraisal process.

What counts towards CPD? The Institute of Healthcare Managers (www.ihm.org.uk) list 10 main types of activity. We think they are comprehensive and about as good as it comes:

- formal study
- work-related
- action learning
- networking
- personal growth and development
- mentoring
- secondment
- experiential learning/self-taught
- attending events
- external learning.

☑ The amount of CPD that staff can be expected to undertake will depend upon on their individual development needs, and may vary from year to year.

☺

Every health professional is responsible for the quality of their service. CPD is a means of achieving higher standards of service.

☑ To see how this is all working out for GPs, look at *A Review of Continuing Professional Development in General Practice*, a report by none other than the Chief Medical Officer. You can find it at: www.publications.doh.gov.uk/pub/docs/doh/cmodev.pdf.

Continuing professional development is a key element in providing a quality service. Don't believe us? Look out HSC 1999/154 *Continuing professional development: quality in the new NHS*. This is the foundation document that should be lurking on the shelves someplace in the practice. It spells out the personal and organisational responsibilities for developing CPD. To save you some time, here are the edited highlights!

- Training and development plans should have been in place for most NHS health professional staff by April 2000
- Arrangements for and investments in CPD should be audited.
- A locally managed system of CPD should be developed.
- Team-based and multidisciplinary learning is encouraged, as is linking of individual CPD goals to those of the organisation for which they work.

Here are a few 'to do's

- Identify suitable courses and modules to train staff.
- Fix budgets, budget heads and budget holders.
- Appoint CPD manager/s with responsibilities for staff within staff groups, service areas and – if the practice is in more than one place – locations.
- Review CPD requirements and learning outcomes.

☺ How would you arrange these types of CPD activity for your practice:
1 courses, study days, conference, seminars
2 studying for a relevant higher degree or other qualification
3 research activities
4 coaching, tutoring or teaching
5 supervision and training of lower grade staff
6 supervision of students
7 mentoring activities
8 membership of, and active participation in, organisations relevant to the member of staff's own field of interest
9 review of articles/books plus presentation to peers
10 review of articles/books plus written circulation to peers
11 observational visit plus written summary of learning outcome and application to working practice
12 case presentation to peers
13 presentation of research/small study to peers
14 self-directed study with preset learning objectives
15 short-term goals for specific sessions with a brief summary for each recorded session on learning outcome.

The new GMS contract recognises the importance of practice management and includes a competency framework.

Here is a list of the headings:

1 Care pathways
2 Liaison with secondary/tertiary care providers
3 Strategy formulation
4 Innovation
5 Clinical audit
6 Organisational audit

☺ See, it's a nice long list!

Well worth taking a look at the detail. Eighty-one sections to keep you entertained and all learned-up!

7 Clinical effectiveness (CE)/evidence-based practice (EBP)
8 Resource allocation
9 Professional development
10 Research
11 Health and safety
12 Fire safety
13 Risk assessment
14 Significant event audit/reporting
15 Infection control
16 Confidentiality
17 Ethics
18 Occupational health
19 Poor performance
20 Disaster planning
21 GP time management
22 Locums
23 Partnership meetings
24 Partnership agreement
25 Partnership changes
26 Taxation
27 CPD requirements
28 Reception
29 Information
30 Clinics/health promotion
31 Complaints
32 Community liaison
33 Patient protection
34 Community nursing
35 Social services
36 Working partnership
37 Networking with colleagues from other practices
38 Petty cash
39 Payroll and pensions
40 Invoice payment
41 Insurance
42 Monthly accounting
43 Annual accounts Claims/targets/quality payments
44 Drawings
45 Quarterly statements
46 Bank and accountant

47 Cash flow/budgets
48 Staff funding
49 Planning
50 information
51 Service budgets
52 Deficiency register
53 Resource negotiation
54 Staff management
55 Staff meetings
56 Rotas and work
57 Recruitment and selection
58 Induction and training

. . . and
59 Employment practice
60 Disciplinary and grievance
61 Performance review
62 Pastoral care
63 Supplies
64 Equipment
65 Facilities management and maintenance
66 Facilities provision
67 Security
68 Project management equipment/premises
69 Patient records
70 Data management
71 Data security
72 Data interpretation/manipulation
73 Hardware maintenance
74 GP links
75 Crisis management
76 Project management
77 Health needs assessment
78 Service performance indicators
79 Strategic delivery planning
80 Service prioritisation
81 Resource negotiation.

Need more?

CPD is now NHS-wide and a million miles deep. Too much of it for a section in a book. These are just the basics. For more detailed advice, that is discipline-specific, click your way to:

- Association of Medical Secretaries, Practice Managers, Administrators and Receptionists (AMSPAR): www.amspar.co.uk
- Institute of Healthcare Management (IHM): www.ihm.org.uk
- National Association of Primary Care (NAPC): www.primarycare.co.uk
- National Primary Care Collaborative (NPCC): www.npdt.org/scripts/default.asp?site_id=5
- National Primary Care Development Team (NPCDT): www.npdt.org/scripts/default.asp?site_id=21
- Royal College of General Practitioners (RCGP): www.rcgp.org.uk
- Royal College of Nursing: www.rcn.org.uk.

CLINICAL NEGLIGENCE

Clinical negligence is a term that is used to mean poor clinical practice of an unacceptable standard. It is, in fact, alleged **wrongdoing** in the area of expertise of a practitioner and may be challenged by the injured party in **civil** law.

Allegations of negligence may be made against a GP and if made and refuted, can be judged in court.

It is possible to raise proceedings against a GP under **tort**, which is interpersonal wrongdoing short of criminality. Action may also be taken under the **law of contract**, which deals with disputes arising from legally enforceable agreements.

For negligence to be demonstrated there is a requirement to be able to demonstrate that:

> ☢ If a GP injures one of their patients and it is unquestionably their fault and they should have realised the risk when they did the treatment. A claim for negligence against them is almost bound to succeed and the insurer will want to settle it as quickly and cheaply as possible.

- the practitioner owed a duty of care to the person making the claim
- that the duty of care was breached
- that an injury was suffered
- that the injury was the direct result of the breach of the duty of care (known as causation)
- that the injury was foreseeable.

In addition, claims arising in **private practice** may be generated by alleged breach of contract as well as by negligence.

> ☑ All of these elements must be demonstrable if the claimant is to succeed in an allegation of negligence.

A **contract** is an agreement creating obligations that are recognised and enforceable by law.

For there to be a contract there must be:

- an offer
- an acceptance
- a consideration – the price (payment) for which the contract is bought.

> ✍ These arrangements only apply to private practice. For work carried out under the NHS, no **consideration** passes between the NHS patient and the treatment practitioner or hospital.

THE DUTY OF CARE

The duty of care is the professional obligation that a GP has to a patient and is enshrined in common law. Such a duty exists from the point at which a patient is accepted explicitly or implicitly.

It is usually clear-cut although there are circumstances where the GP may find that his or her primary duty is to someone other than the patient. For example, a GP may be asked to write a report on a patient's condition for an insurance company or an employer. In such a circumstance the GP–patient relationship does not exist in conventional terms but the GP does still have a duty to comply with professional requirements and to avoid causing harm.

In negligence cases the practitioner has to demonstrate that what he or she did was appropriate and of an adequate standard. This is achieved by a judicial review of professional opinion to assess **the standard of care**.

In other words, a practitioner cannot act in a certain way in the absolute knowledge that his or her actions could not subsequently be challenged and an allegation of negligence made.

In 1957 the pivotal *Bolam* case (*Bolam* v *Friern Hospital Management Committee*) established the essence of negligence by setting the standard for a breach of duty of care.

The standard set was of the ordinarily skilled man exercising and professing to have that special skill. The man did not need to possess the highest expert skill in order to avoid being found guilty of negligence. For the law it was sufficient for him to exercise the ordinary skill of the ordinary competent man exercising that particular art.

The *Bolam* judgement followed a case two years earlier in Scotland when Lord President Clyde set out the definition for medical negligence in the case of *Hunter* v *Hanley*. He said:

> 'The true test for establishing negligence and diagnosis or treatment on the part of the doctor is whether he has been proved to be guilty of such failure as no doctor of ordinary skill would be guilty of if acting with ordinary care.'

He later expanded this view by stating that:

> '. . . liability could be established only with the demonstration of three factors; firstly that there is a normal and usual practice, secondly that the doctor had not adopted that practice and thirdly that the course the doctor adopted is one that no professional man of ordinary skill would have taken.'

Both in Scotland and England these judgements related to a negligence allegation involving a medical practitioner but the judgements have been rolled out across the whole spectrum of healthcare.

The clear message that emanates from these two cases is that acting reasonably to the standard of your peers provides a defence against an allegation of negligence.

Part of the success in a case of alleged negligence (in those cases that reach court) is that the experts impress the judge as being honest and reasonable.

This factor was very important in a further case that has influenced negligence cases; the *Bolitho* case (*Bolitho and others* v *City and Hackney Health Authority 1997*). This was a complicated case that went to the Court of Appeal and ultimately to the House of Lords and led to consideration of the issues surrounding the situation where experts acting for both sides both offered compelling arguments.

A judge normally relies on the clinical evidence in order to make a judgement and in such circumstances, he has to decide whether the experts acting for the claimant or the defendant submitted the more logical and sustainable arguments. In fact, in this case, the judges ultimately found for the defendant but the case laid down important criteria. It reinforced the paramount status of the *Bolam* case and *Hunter* v *Hanley*. It also made clear that experts must be of the highest calibre and able to carefully consider the issues and articulate their views on a convincing basis.

In essence, *Bolitho*, whilst upholding the test of reasonableness, reminded the professions that, in circumstances where there is expert opinion on both sides, the judge must decide which body of opinion is more reasonable and convincing.

The **standard of proof** required in a civil case is that a particular event was more likely than not to have happened, i.e. the balance of probabilities as opposed to the criminal standard, which is beyond reasonable doubt.

Causation is a term used to describe whether an incident (through act or omission) if alleged to be negligent, actually caused or materially contributed, to a loss or injury. If a GP provides treatment and there is an adverse outcome, but it can be shown that the outcome would have been the same irrespective of whether the treatment had been provided, then the GP cannot be held to be negligent.

Some commentators' views, based on the *Bolam* and *Hunter* v *Hanley* judgements, regard the negligence situation as biased in favour of healthcare practitioners. They see as difficult the fact that the claimant (pursuer in Scotland) has to prove that the practitioner (defendant in England and Wales or defender in Scotland) who breached the duty of care, specifically caused or contributed to the loss or injury in circumstances that were reasonably foreseeable and needs only to act to a reasonable standard of an ordinarily skilled practitioner, rather than someone practising to the best standard possible. Many practitioners, particularly those who have been accused of negligence may well say that things are difficult enough as they are.

Compensation for an injury in a civil claim can only be by the payment of money. Successful claimants are usually awarded **general** and **special** damages. Such settlements may be 'once-and-for-all' payments although they may be staged over a period of time, up to and including the lifetime of the recipient.

These payments are not entirely without conditions. A claimant has a duty to mitigate the loss. In other words, if a claimant suffers an injury at the hands of a GP and appropriate corrective treatment may reduce or resolve the consequences or the suffering, then the treatment should not be delayed until the outcome of the trial is known, or settlement reached, before receiving the treatment in question.

If a claimant refuses treatment that could have lessened the duration or consequences of the injury, then the claimant must demonstrate that his refusal to accept the treatment was reasonable.

General damages are awarded for the pain and suffering associated with the injury suffered. **Special damages** are awarded as a specific payment especially for the claimant's particular injury and the consequences that are the result of the injury. The damages may be calculated on a range of factors.

Much of the claim will be associated with the costs associated with any immediate corrective treatment and any costs associated with further treatment that would be required in the future. However, other costs that can be added are such things as radiology, drug costs, travel costs and expert opinion paid for by the claimant and even appliances.

In a circumstance, for example, where a GP has injured a patient and the treatment of the injury required some sort of individually prepared equipment, the equipment would be expected to wear out and the special damages would include a calculation based on the replacement cycle of the device, the person's life expectancy and the expected future cost of the device.

A calculation is performed that should arrive at a lump sum which, when invested, would be expected to provide for the treatment costs over the claimant's lifetime.

In successful cases claimants are also entitled to receive interest on damages awarded, calculated from the date of the clinical incident giving rise to the claim.

> ☢ Claimants are entitled to the costs of **private** corrective treatment even though the same treatment might be available under the National Health Service.

Compensation recovery may be influenced by the nature of the injury sustained. If the claimant has received state benefits as a result of the alleged injury, then these payments will be deducted from the eventual compensation by the **Compensation Recovery Unit**.

In the case of a serious injury, in circumstances where the claimant is paid considerable compensation in excess of that allowed for capital holdings with certain means-tested benefits, he or she may not be able to receive those state benefits until their means dwindle. It is possible to circumvent this problem by placing the compensation in a special needs trust fund with the claimant as the only beneficiary.

Time for a lie down in a dark room, or perhaps a cuppa?

THE PROCESS OF THE LAW

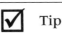

Tip

The Civil Procedure Rules apply to England and Wales but NOT to Scotland

The litigation process underwent a huge change following a review of the previous procedure by Lord Woolf, who was appointed to do so by the Lord Chancellor in 1994. The new Civil Procedure Rules came into effect in 1998. Their purposes were:

- to improve access to justice
- to reduce the costs of litigation
- to reduce the complexity of the rules
- to remove outmoded and outdated terminology
- to bring consistency to the process.

Lord Woolf's key objective was to ensure that courts were enabled to deal with cases justly, by trying to place the parties on an equal footing, saving expense and dealing with the case in ways proportionate to the amount of money involved, the importance of the case and its complexity. He also wanted to see cases dealt with expeditiously and with an appropriate amount of court time.

In the **legal process** patients will generally instruct a solicitor who specialises in clinical negligence cases. Some claimants bring a case themselves and they are known as '**litigants in person**'. This brave band has often achieved stunning success because the court may help them to achieve a fair outcome, even though their inexperience may cause confusion to all involved in the court process.

Legal costs may be considerable in some cases involving GPs. The general position in the UK is that the loser in a case pays the costs of the winner. If a claimant discontinues a case once court proceedings have been issued then he or she is also responsible for the opposing GP's costs.

It is only when a claimant is legally aided that he or she is not generally responsible for the GP's costs, if unsuccessful. Legal costs may be substantial, running into many thousands of pounds. GPs must be indemnified against claims for negligence. The insurer should provide advice and support at an in-house level, should provide legal representation for the GP at any court hearing and should deal with all correspondence so that the GP is not troubled by direct contact from the claimant's solicitor. The insurer should pay all applicable legal costs and any compensation awarded by a court or agreed in a settlement.

When a claimant sets out to take action against a GP, a solicitor is normally instructed. The claimant must decide how the claim will be funded and there are several possibilities:

- **Legal Aid, also known as public funding:** This is now becoming much harder to obtain following recent changes to the rules governing eligibility.
- **Legal expenses insurance:** Many claimants have this sort of insurance as part of their household buildings and contents policies. Such policies pay the costs of an unsuccessful claim.

With both Legal Aid and legal expenses insurance, claimants will not be liable for costs if the case is lost and there is therefore little risk in bringing a claim.

- **Private funding of a claim:** Some claimants fund their own claims but the huge potential costs of significant claims may act as an effective deterrent in such circumstances.
- **Conditional fee agreements:** Also known as 'no-win, no-fee' agreements, they are backed by insurance

> ✍ **Make a note**
> The fee for access to the Health records is £10 and it is recommended that photocopies are charged at 33 pence a sheet (maximum £50).

policies to pay the legal costs if the case is lost. Furthermore, a claimant's solicitor may receive a **success fee** if the case is won. The court can order the success fee and the insurance premium to be paid as additional legal costs if the claimant wins the case.

The process usually starts with the solicitor obtaining details of the proposed claim and the circumstances surrounding the alleged negligence. An investigation is then launched by the solicitor to assess the merits of the allegation. A request will be made to the GP for the release of the clinical records.

☑ If you receive such a request then you should notify your defence, medico-legal adviser immediately. He or she will help you to deal with the request.

Records must be provided within 40 days and there is a standard (small) fee payable for providing them together with a fee per page of notes copied. The solicitor may also seek medical records from any other healthcare professional or hospital involved.

A request for records does not automatically mean that a negligence claim will follow. In many cases a review of the records may demonstrate that the GP operated in a completely appropriate or professional way.

The assessment may be made by the solicitor but frequently the opinion of an expert is sought, to review the available information and to evaluate the merits of the case. The initial assessment is vitally important for the funding arrangements. If the report is not supportive of the claimant's contention, then the Legal Aid Board or a prospective 'after the event' insurer will not be prepared to fund the case.

If the expert opinion offers a **reasonable prospect of success**, the case may proceed to the next stage. A **letter of claim** is sent to the GP or to the insurer representing the GP if known.

The letter of claim sets out the claimant's case in as much detail as possible. It contains a description of the alleged facts, the main allegations of alleged negligence, a description of the injuries that the claimant suffered, the diagnosis and prognosis with a description of the remedial treatment and any likely residual damage.

The letter also explains the **causation** (i.e. how the claimant contributed to or caused the injury alleged) and gives details of the damages sought (the financial claim made). From the letter of claim the GP and the defence organisation advisers should be able to understand the detail of the claim and enable a full investigation so that the GP can answer the allegations.

Generally the GP's advisers will also acquire full copies of all relevant records and any statements necessary to assist in the assessment. The GP will be interviewed by claims staff and/or a solicitor, acting for the insurer and his or her recollections of events carefully questioned.

Assistance may be obtained by engaging an expert to give an initial opinion on the merits of the case. This will enable the insurer to assess whether it is defensible or whether an offer to settle the matter should be negotiated. The insurer will then enter into discussion with the GP about the overall impression of the claim and will seek agreement on the best way to handle it.

> ☑ The civil procedure rules provide for a 90-day period within which the letter of claim should be answered.

Within the letter of claim the claimant may include an **offer to settle** (also known as a **Part 36 offer**). This sets out the amount that he or she would be prepared to accept to settle the claim.

This offer has important implications if it is rejected and the case continues but the claim is finally settled for a sum equal to or less than that made in the original offer – the court could take the view that the initial offer should have been accepted and it will impose a penalty when assessing the award of legal costs at the conclusion of the case.

The GP and the defence advisory team have 90 days to consider the letter of claim, to undertake the necessary research and to construct a full response. It is hoped that, by going through this procedure, the issues will have been identified and the case resolved without the need for costly and often stressful litigation.

In general the outcome of the investigations will result in one of the following responses:

- A rebuttal of the allegation.
- An acknowledgement of the injuries and an agreement to settle the claim as made by the claimant.
- Recognition of a degree of culpability and a counteroffer to settle on behalf of the GP. For example, the claimant might seek £50 000 and the GP offer to settle for £20 000. As with any offer made by the claimant, there would be cost consequences for the claimant if the GP's offer was rejected and in the final settlement the same or a lesser amount was accepted.

Limitation is the term used to describe the point beyond which claimants lose the right to issue proceedings. The law as it currently stands in England and Wales sets the limitation period at the third anniversary of the date on which the incident occurred or the third anniversary of the date from which the claimant became aware that an injury had been suffered.

In general, for children below the age of 18, they have until they reach 18 plus three years to make a claim. A GP may therefore experience a claim many years after an incident occurred.

Experts are employed to evaluate the clinical management of the GP and to make an assessment of the claim and decide whether the GP's actions constituted negligence.

The *Bolam* test really creates the notion of peer review as the means of assessing the GP's work. When a claimant approaches a solicitor, the solicitor may, as part of his review of the claim, seek initial expert opinion, as may the defence insurer when in receipt of the letter of claim.

> ☢ Both sides may obtain an expert opinion although the court has the power to instruct both sides to use the same expert.

If the claim is disputed, further expert opinion will be required. Both sides may obtain an expert opinion although the court has the power to instruct both sides to use the same expert.

The expert will be provided with detailed instructions by the court and they will be made available to both sides. The expert must be careful to report only within his or her own area of expertise. The expert's duty is to **inform the court** irrespective of who engages his or her services. The opinion should be independent and should not conceal evidence that might assist the other party.

If the case is not resolved at the pre-action stage, then the claimant must decide whether to issue court proceedings. The GP's response to the letter of claim will have made clear whether the insurers had decided that there was no claim to answer.

If there is a rebuttal and the claimant decides to proceed with the claim, then he or she will have to issue a **claim form**. This is an official court document that lays out the detail of the claim and must have with it an expert report substantiating the claim and a schedule giving the details of the damages sought. Once the claim form is issued at a court it must be served on the GP within a prescribed time (four months). The GP is now referred to as a defendant.

Once the claim form has been served the GP has 28 days to serve a defence, which must fully address all the allegations and the issues contained within the claim form. Once the defence is served, the court will send out questionnaires to both parties to enquire about the number of witnesses and experts that they each intend to call. The court will also explore the possibility of a **stay of proceedings** to give the parties the opportunity to see whether they can settle the case without recourse to court.

Once all the paperwork is complete the judge will consider all the documents and decide how to manage the case.

The court track is a term used to describe the route through the court system for any individual case. Essentially claims worth less than £5000 go through the **small claims** court, claims worth less than £15 000 and suitable for a one-day hearing go through the **fast track** and all other cases go through the **multi-track route**.

> You can't keep secret some documents and in a Perry Mason-esque way announce them at the trial to make the other side's case collapse.
>
> Evidence cannot generally be introduced at trial if it has not been exchanged in accordance with court direction.

The multi-track is the most likely route for GP cases. Depending on the value and complexity of the case it may be heard in a High Court rather than a county court.

The judge will schedule a case conference to agree a timetable for the case leading to trial. It will also be used as an opportunity to identify areas of agreement between the parties and therefore limit the areas of dispute. Judges have wide powers in these circumstances and therefore may make a variety of decisions depending on their perspective of the case.

Preparation for trial

Once the timetable is agreed, both parties must exchange all relevant documents to the other side. These will generally include all clinical records, all correspondence, all statements and any invoices incurred by the patient as part of the costs identified for the special damages claim. This process is designed to ensure that both parties have all the relevant information available to them.

Legal privilege

Correspondence between a lawyer and his client need not be disclosed to the other side because it attracts legal privilege. This protection extends to the advisers involved in the case.

Witness statements

These are generally exchanged at the same time by both sides. The statements will have described the events as recollected by the witnesses. They may not only include the GP and the claimant but also such people as receptionists, colleagues, relatives of the claimant and hospital staff and anyone else who was involved.

At a later stage, both sides exchange expert witness reports. This then enables each side to discover, consider and appreciate the strengths and weaknesses of the other side's arguments. Once these reports have been seen, it is not uncommon for the parties to agree a settlement.

Once proceedings have been issued the defendant can make a **payment into court** additional to any offer to settle made in the letter of response. If the defendant or the advisers decide on this course of action it is paid into the court office. The claimant has 21 days to consider the offer. As with any previous offer, if the claimant refuses the payment as inadequate and the court subsequently awards the same or less in damages there is a considerable penalty in that the claimant would be responsible for paying his and the defendant's legal costs from 21 days after the payment was made.

At **trial** the judge, who will not have been involved in previous case management, will not be aware of any payments made into court. There is no jury. The case will be open to the public and to journalists. Cases involving GPs, particularly if there is any salacious element, may attract a lot of journalistic interest. Both claimant and defendant will each be represented by a barrister whom they will have met and with whom they will previously have had a conference.

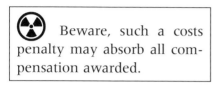 Beware, such a costs penalty may absorb all compensation awarded.

In the United Kingdom judicial system the court procedure is **adversarial**. It can be a most unpleasant experience and everyone giving evidence will experience it.

Each witness will be questioned by his or her own barrister and then be cross-examined by the barrister acting for the other side. A similar process will occur with expert witnesses and other witnesses for both sides. The judge, too, may ask questions to clarify the facts.

At the end of the case the barristers for the claimant and the GP (defendant) will make closing speeches. After everything has been presented the judge will consider all the evidence and give a **judgement**.

The judgement may be given orally or in a written judgement some time after the conclusion of the case. If the claimant is successful, then the compensation must be paid within a short time. The winner's legal costs are, by convention, paid by the losing party. However, it is not uncommon for the judge **not** to award costs against a claimant if they lose, presumably because of awareness that the GP is defended by an insurance company.

If either party is dissatisfied with the judgement, either party may appeal. For the practitioner an appeal is a serious step. It is expensive, and so an insurer will not support it unless there is a reasonable prospect of success. To fail at appeal will add to adverse publicity in many cases. Any doctor wishing to appeal a decision should discuss the matter in detail with the defence insurer legal adviser to establish whether grounds actually exist for doing so.

The whole process of a claim is unpleasant and distressing. The insurance medico-legal adviser should provide support and assistance and is often friend, confidante and ally as well as adviser. Data is very variable but reassuringly, about three-quarters of all claims come to nothing and only about 1 in 20 actually finds its way into court.

☑ Tip

GPs may be asked for a report about a patient and the treatment provided. The solicitor's letter may contain a sentence such as 'No action is contemplated against you in this matter' or 'There is no suggestion that your treatment is under scrutiny'.

GPs wonder whether this is an indemnity against ending up in court if it is subsequently decided that the GP does have some sort of case to answer.

The answer is that, subject to time limits, the GP can be joined, later, in a legal action if information suggesting negligence comes to light. The solicitor cannot indemnify the GP because he or she cannot be sure that more information may not subsequently emerge.

Advice: before agreeing to give a statement, contact your insurance company medico-legal adviser and obtain advice about what you should say in a statement.

THE TELEPHONE: GETTING WIRED

Good communication is often the difference between success and failure in a consultation. Increasingly, consultations are occurring on the telephone. The doctor is required to take a history, carry out a verbal examination, make some sort of working diagnosis and suggest treatment or further management without ever seeing the patient.

This is no small task and carries with it the inherent risk of failure to diagnose because of misunderstanding the patient or misrepresentation of the symptoms.

Furthermore, patients may feel that the telephone is merely a way of being fobbed off without receiving a home visit or a surgery consultation.

Clinicians often feel that it is not possible to do an adequate assessment of a patient without seeing him or her. The Department of Health seems to believe that it can be done.

The culture of healthcare has changed, NHS Direct and NHS 24 in Scotland are well established and doctors are increasingly expected to work in this way. So, here are a few tips to ensure that your telephone experience provides the lowest risk for you and your patient.

REVIEWING THE PRACTICE SYSTEM

The first thing to do is to stand back and review your telephone system. We often telephone surgeries – some answering arrangements are excellent whilst others are, well, frankly dreadful.

Not many of us have the time to listen to seven options, three of which involve hanging up and telephoning another number. We generally don't want to listen to several minutes of 'Greensleeves'. We certainly don't want to be confronted by a receptionist who says, 'Good morning, Surgery. Hold on . . .' and then places you on hold for what seems like an eternity without giving you any sort of opportunity to say why you are telephoning or whether it is convenient to wait.

> ☑ Put some 10 pence pieces into your pocket and walk down the road to the telephone box. Ring your surgery and see how good your service is. You might find yourself rushing back to change something – or somebody!

Remember that the better the telephone system, the less likely a patient is to be dissatisfied with the subsequent communication.

MAKING CONTACT

When a patient telephones and speaks to a member of the practice staff, the first thing that happens is the **verbal handshake**. Is it firm and confident or weak and wobbly?

> ☺ Aim to ensure the telephone is answered within five rings.

TELEPHONE CONSULTATION?

Remember, the conversation isn't just for the practitioner to make an assessment of the patient. The patient will generally have made an assessment of the doctor within 30 seconds and will have decided whether they are someone they can 'do business' with.

> ☢ If you really are under pressure and you have to do something else, tell the patient that you **do** want to speak with them and that you will ring them back (say) in 20 minutes. If you say you will, **do it or die in the attempt!** Don't be stampeded into action – you'll regret it.

If they've decided that the doc doesn't know what they are doing or that they are not going to listen to them or examine them in the way that they want, then the doc might just as well be talking to themselves. The conversation or consultation will be doomed to failure.

Let us assume that the GP's first interaction with the patient is excellent and they have given the impression that they are Doctors Findlay, Kildare, Quincy and every other wonderful television doctor all rolled into one.

☺ THIS NEXT BIT IS FOR THE GPS

If you are going to do a telephone consultation there is a lot to remember:

1 **Don't sound rushed:** However busy you are, sound as though you have all the time in the world and it is all for the patient. If you sound as though you are in a hurry the patient will realise and the outcome of the conversation will be less satisfactory and is real ammunition if the tele-consult goes wrong.

2 **Be sympathetic:** Disinterested is bad news and lacking in sympathy is even worse. For you it may just be another sore throat; for the patient it is the symptom that has prevented him or her going to work, singing in the choir or making a career-building presentation. The last thing they want is for you not to show any interest. Fail and the consultation will fall apart!

3 **Listen!** Patients want to tell you all about their problems. Now we understand that eventually you might have to interrupt, but doctors seem incapable of keeping quiet for more than a few seconds before the urge to interrupt overcomes them. The more you interrupt, the less successful the consultation will be. If the conversation starts to ramble, steer it rather than stopping it.

4 **Try some 'active listening':** If you do listen without making any sounds at all, such that the patient interrupts themselves to see if you are still there or if you have gone to sleep, the consultation will go less well. Adopt a policy of active listening – throw in an occasional 'yes', 'ah ha', 'OK', 'mmmmm', and so on, to indicate that you are alive. Consider saying to the patient, 'Just hold on a second whilst I write a note of this'. It confirms you are listening with a purpose.

5 **If you have questions to ask to help you reach a diagnosis, tell the patient why you are asking them.** Being confronted by questions may confuse the patient and may sound very like a ploy to avoid actually seeing them. So, explain why the answers will help you to make the correct assessment.

6 **Finally**, make sure you actually understand what you have been told. Repeat back the important elements of the information so that there is no doubt in anyone's mind that everything has been understood.

WHAT ABOUT THE ANGRY OR DIFFICULT PATIENT?

Remember the five golden rules:

1 **Don't hang up on the caller:** You have two problems then! You have to recover from hanging up and re-establish the relationship.
2 **If you *have* to go**, stop the call by explaining the reason and confirming that you **will** call back – and do so, or die!
3 **Let bad language and shouting pass you by:** Some people do not agree with this advice and clearly there will be times when you do need to challenge an abusive caller. However, in general, if you respond to aggression with calmness and ignore rude comments, the likelihood is that the caller will calm down, abandon aggressive language and run out of steam.
4 **Speak slowly, quietly and calmly:** If the caller gets agitated, it is easy to up the pace of the dialogue. Try to respond slowly, quietly and calmly. However, do everything to avoid sounding patronising – there is nothing more likely to inflame a situation!

And . . .

> ☑ Never make an important phone call sitting down. We don't know why it works – it just does. Something about transmitting body language down the phone. Anyway, try it for yourself!

5 **If you are wrong, say so.**

Handling people on the telephone is an art, and however good you are at it, you will not get it right every time. However, to complete a telephone call with a satisfied customer is well worthwhile and the feeling of relief when an annoyed caller goes away satisfied is priceless.

Examining and Treating the Patient

Compared to examining and treating a patient, all other risks are a walk in the park! In this respect patients come with a happy bundle of threats and risks!

Whenever a patient enters the surgery you have no idea whether the subsequent consultation will go well or badly, whether you will make a correct diagnosis, whether an error will haunt you for ages or whether some other event or incident will cause you and the patient distress.

> ☺ Cheer up! The vast majority of consultations go really well. The outcome is usually delighted patients and GPs who are happy that their professional standards have been met.

But – and it is a big but . . .

There is no intent in this chapter to tell you how to examine or treat the patient. Your professional skills are a matter for you, your patients, your PCT and in extreme cases, the GMC! And, if you are really wicked, you might get a day or two in London, at the Law Courts in the Strand.

The purpose of this section is to draw attention to known risks and pitfalls that have caught out practitioners in the past in the hope that a bell might ring if you find yourself in a similar situation.

Prevention, they say, is better than cure, and GPs who have found themselves on the wrong side of the GMC professional conduct committee or a negligence allegation would wholeheartedly agree.

> Remember: no notes, no defence
> We know it has been said before but it can't be said too often!

Here's the fundamental: GPs have to act reasonably. That means under-taking the elements of an examination and providing treatment that would be regarded as normal practice by a reasonable body of your ordinarily skilled colleagues.

And don't forget that the notes have to show that you did it.

The process of examining and treating a patient has several components. Let's consider the risks under the following headings:

- appearances
- taking the history
- doing the examination
- providing the treatment.

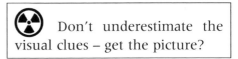 Medico-legal reviews indicate that GPs often fail to recognise pallor, oedema, signs of cardiac failure and jaundice.

APPEARANCES

Appearances, as they say, can be deceptive. But you can learn a lot from appearances. Some errors occur because GPs just do not look at their patients. Observation should be a key element of examination. In concentrating on the specific issue of concern to the patient at that particular consultation, the GP can miss straightforward medical signs. The best examination will integrate the two approaches.

Medical studies indicate just how important appearance actually is. The information gleaned from a non-physical examination can be divided into what you see and what you hear.

The studies suggest that over half of all information is gained from looking at the patient; the way he or she walks, sits down, moves, gesticulates, the body language in general, as well as more general factors such as dress and more specific medical factors such as the presence of peripheral oedema, breathlessness, colour and clubbing.

Don't underestimate the visual clues – get the picture?

HISTORY

History often provides vital clues that assist in diagnosis and govern the treatments which may be provided. Allegations of negligence not uncommonly arise from failure to take an adequate history. A review of cases suggests that previous malignancy and details of therapeutic drug usage may be missed.

> ☢ Every year there are medico-legal catastrophes associated with a failure to identify known allergies.

THE EXAMINATION

The examination builds on the information gleaned in the history and enables the GP to reach a diagnosis. Examination is clearly a fundamental part of the treatment planning and allegations of poor professional standards and negligence indicate that, on occasion, GPs do forget important elements of the examination.

The following common pitfalls in general practice form a large part of the claims made against GPs and although not in any particular order, they should make a practitioner think twice when confronted with any one.

1 **Missed malignancy:** The most common claim against GPs relates to missed malignancies in general. Of those, three are the most noteworthy:

   a **Colon:** About 4% of the population will suffer carcinoma of the colon and an average GP will see two or three new cases every year. The symptoms and signs that are often missed should never be taken lightly. Watch out for:

   - passage of blood or mucus
   - constipation or change in bowel habit in someone with previously regular bowel action, especially if of cancer age.

   If you see them, do not dismiss them as piles or lack of roughage.

   The patient will need lower bowel studies such as sigmoidoscopy, colonoscopy or barium enema.

   GPs should **not** make a new diagnosis of irritable bowel syndrome on the basis of pain, wind or change of bowel habit at any age. IBS is a diagnosis of exclusion.

b **Brain:** Headache is a very common symptom and brain tumours are rare, occurring only in about five people per 100 000 per year. Most tumours are secondary. An average GP is likely to see a patient with a brain tumour only once every eight to 10 years. For the GP there is a major dilemma. Refer every headache and face the wrath of the local neurologist whose clinic you will block up, or risk missing a brain tumour. Clearly the judgement has to be based on a careful history, the location of the headache, associated symptoms and examination of the fundi. Headaches, particularly if there are any symptoms causing any concern whatsoever, should be carefully documented in the notes and the reason for reaching the diagnosis carefully explained.

c **Breast:** The commonest cancer in women, there is approximately a one in 15 chance that a woman will develop the disease. Breast lumps are common in the surgery and each should be very carefully assessed. GPs should not be diverted from performing a proper examination by embarrassment or reassurance from the patient that 'they often come and go' or 'aren't anything really'. Examination alone is not sufficient to make a judgement that a discrete breast lump is benign. Unless it disappears completely the patient should be referred for investigation, and probably for excision of the lump and histology.

2 **Meningitis:** About 2% of claims against GPs relate to failed diagnosis of meningitis but represent a substantial part of damages awards paid by defence organisations, particularly in those cases where an individual is left with a handicap.

> Anyone who has been criticised for failure to diagnose meningitis will understand just how difficult it is. Indeed, some authorities say that any doctor who has not been caught out by an early meningitis has simply been lucky!

The early symptoms of meningitis are often those of a self-limiting viral illness and the classical features do not appear until later in the course of the illness. Those doctors who are accused of missing the diagnosis and who are exonerated are frequently defended by the quality of their notes.

In any case where there is **any suspicion** of meningitis, the patient should be admitted for lumbar puncture and penicillin (unless contra-indicated) should be commenced **immediately**. In cases where there is even the remotest possibility that the symptoms could evolve into a meningitis, the patient or the family should be carefully briefed on what to look out for and if possible, given a leaflet about meningitis.

3 **Gynaecological errors:**

   a **Ectopic pregnancy:** Easy to miss, particularly in its early stages, the number of incidents is rising and failure to make the diagnosis is causing a rise in the number of negligence claims.

   The classical symptoms of pain, bleeding and a brown vaginal discharge with a history of a missed period are straightforward but, alas, the presentation is often nothing like so simple. If there is any suspicion of an ectopic pregnancy the patient should be referred immediately to hospital for a pregnancy test and an ultrasound scan. It is a diagnosis to be considered in any woman of child-bearing age with symptoms below the chest and above the knees.

   b **Contraceptive problems:** Any contraception can fail and GPs should not be lulled into a false sense of security in respect of the possibility of pregnancy simply because the woman was using some form of contraception. In particular there should be particular attention to:

   • low abdominal symptoms in women with intrauterine contraceptive devices

   • drug interactions with oral contraceptives. In particular, failures of oral contraceptives associated with the use of antibiotics or anti-convulsants with ensuing pregnancies where no warnings were given (and written in the patient notes!) may lead to expensive claims.

4 **Appendicitis:** Still a condition that results in missed diagnosis and claims against GPs. Although the incidence appears to be declining it should always be another diagnosis considered in the 'below the waist' symptoms experienced by patients at any age.

5 **Chest pain:** Patients complaining of pain in the chest present a recurring and regular diagnostic problem for GPs. The use of clinical acumen to differentiate between pain in the chest emanating from the heart, chest wall, upper gastrointestinal tract or lungs/pleura is an important skill but it may be very risky to use clinical skills alone unless the diagnosis is absolutely clear.

   And, even then . . . The risk of development of a dysrhythmia and sudden death should always be at the back of the mind and litigation may well follow a death in cases where cardiac chest pain had formerly been dismissed.

   It goes without saying that a careful assessment of any patient is essential and the notes should reflect the consideration of the differential diagnosis. Judges, at negligence trials, are unimpressed by entries in medical notes that say:

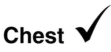

Chest ✓

6 **Subarachnoid haemorrhage:** This is another diagnosis that GPs should consider themselves lucky not to have missed. It is not very common in general practice and the average GP can expect to see one only once every three to five years.

However, they are of huge import and the suspicion of a GP should be raised in any patient with a headache or cerebral localising symptoms with a family history, hypertension polycys-

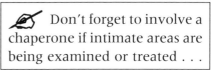 Don't forget to involve a chaperone if intimate areas are being examined or treated . . .

tic kidneys or coarctation of the aorta. The severity of the headache and its suddenness of onset may also be a key clue. Subarachnoid haemorrhages resulting in severe disability may give rise to large negligence claims where the diagnosis is delayed.

During the examination it is extremely important to maintain the patient's modesty, allowing the removal of clothing behind a suitable screen and providing a towel or dressing gown to cover any personal areas. An allegation of voyeurism or worse can damage or destroy a career.

Only necessary clothing should be removed, bearing in mind the balance between good access to areas that need examining and the modesty of the patient. Before examination, make sure that you tell the patient what you are going to do with your hands or with any instruments, so that any action you take does not come as a surprise, particularly in an intimate area.

TREATMENT

The whole crux of risk can be focused on clinical treatment. GPs need to be consistently vigilant and to provide only those therapies for which they are trained and in which they are competent.

☺ All obvious stuff, but if it was that obvious there would not be claims against practitioners.

At the risk of repeating messages given elsewhere in the book; be sure to consider the following six golden rules before or during treatment of the patient:

1 Have you obtained consent and given adequate explanation?
2 Be careful not to mishandle the patient either by word or deed.

3 Avoid inappropriate comments, particularly at a time when emotional tensions may be running high. Patients may find themselves more undressed for longer periods than patients of other healthcare professionals.

4 Do not fail to assess the reactivity of the patient.

5 Do not ignore feedback from the patient regarding treatment.

> **Do not take inappropriate risks**. You should not go home at the end of the day wondering whether any of the treatment that you provided was either not correct or not safe.

• Remember to reassess treatment. You should be careful not to continue with a treatment without critical review. In such circumstances damage may ensue.

PRESCRIBING ERRORS

Prescribing errors could warrant a whole textbook on their own.

GPs write 1.7 million prescriptions a day! No wonder there is a bit of scope for things to go wrong.

So, what can go wrong?

> A medication error is a preventable error that may cause or lead to inappropriate medication, or use, or patient harm while the medication is in control of a healthcare professional.

> ☺ Costs are rising rapidly and the bill for prescriptions has now exceeded £7 billion a year. The average cost of a prescription item in 1950 was 16p. It is now about £11.00.

• Administrative:
  • wrong patient
  • wrong drug
  • wrong dose or frequency
  • writing the prescription incorrectly.
• Clinical:
  • allergy
  • cosmetic, e.g. photosensitivity, depigmentation
  • side-effects, e.g. bleeding, migraine, rash.

Controlled drugs have assumed much greater importance in terms of their administration since the events surrounding Harold Shipman. If storing controlled drugs in the surgery, the practice **must** have a bound, controlled drugs register with consecutively numbered pages.

Problems arise when a GP prescribes a drug with which he or she is unfamiliar, sometimes under pressure from a hospital consultant who wants to transfer responsibility.

In order to prescribe a drug the GP should:

> ☢ Great care should be taken to ensure that someone (the practice manager or a senior practice nurse?) keeps track of all drugs whether in the practice or in doctors' bags: 'the accountable person'.

• understand its actions and benefits
• be aware of side-effects, interactions and complications
• be aware of alternative drug treatments
• be aware of any monitoring requirements and how to manage any abnormal results
• be familiar with the route of drug delivery.

Unlicensed drugs

If you are undertaking a clinical trial with an unlicensed drug, be sure to:

• ensure that the trial is ethical
• ensure that the company objective is achievable
• understand the protocol
• ensure the patient understands the experimental nature of the drug
• ensure that the patient signs a consent form
• check that there is a system for abandoning the trial if concerns arise.

Prescribing outside the licence

GPs may prescribe in this way in circumstances, for example, where a drug is licensed for adults but not for children. In such circumstances the GP must make sure that:

• all concerned understand the side-effects
• parents and/or guardians understand the nature of the drug and the reasons for its use
• a signed consent is obtained from someone with parental responsibility
• they appreciate that the benefits of protection under the Consumer Protection Act is lost.

Repeat prescribing

A large number of errors are associated with repeat prescribing. All practices should have a repeat prescribing policy. All staff should be trained to comply with repeat prescribing requirements.

You should try to ensure that:

- there is a medication sheet on the front of every set of notes
- prescribing should be reviewed at least annually (six monthly is better):
  - Is it still required?
  - Is it most appropriate?
  - Is the dose right?
  - Is it being monitored properly?
  - Has the patient got instruction leaflets?

> ☢ Remember, **the doctor who signs the prescription has the clinical responsibility for its use**. Even if it is a repeat prescription produced on a computer by a receptionist, the same principle applies. So docs: check what you sign. Everyone else, don't get grumpy if the doc appears over-cautious.

CUTTING THE RISK OUT OF SURGERY

Doctors would soon find the practice of medicine pretty boring if all they did was to look at colds and coughs all day.

One way to add a bit of variety is to do some minor surgery in the practice! And the patients like it too. It cuts down waiting times, it is convenient and the patients are treated by someone they know.

However, there is a downside.

☺ The Gods of Whitehall have tried to spice up the doc's daily life by adding a minefield of diagnoses, codes, quality markers and guidance criteria to make total confusion more likely.

☢ A significant proportion of all complaints and claims made against GPs relate to issues associated with minor surgery. Many of them are easily avoidable with a bit of sensible planning.

What is required is a simple risk management strategy!

💡 **Principles of risk management**

1 **Identify the risk:** What can go wrong?
2 **Analyse the risk:** How likely is it to go wrong and how serious an impact might it have?
3 **Control the risk:** What can you do to reduce or eliminate it or transfer it to someone else?
4 **Cost the risk:** What is the cost of getting it right versus the cost of getting it wrong?

What does it take to do the job well? The Seven Golden Rules:

1 good organisation
2 suitable equipment
3 suitable facilities
4 adequate support
5 good preparation
6 adequate surgical skills
7 comprehensive record keeping.

It all looks very straightforward but it seems to go wrong again and again.

DO YOU KNOW WHAT YOU ARE DOING?

As a surgical practitioner you will need to satisfy yourself that you are competent to perform the procedures in question. These days you will need to produce evidence to show effective training and continuing professional development. But how do you get up to speed?

- referring to texts and photographs
- seeking expert tuition
- observing a consultant
- doing cases under supervision
- agreeing protocols with local surgeons
- organising continuing support and access to advice.

☺ Unfortunately, watching episodes of BBC's Casualty programme on a Saturday night doesn't count!

If something does go wrong you will almost certainly be asked to demonstrate how your competence was acquired. Keep the information up to date in your PDF. OK, so what's a PDF? It is your Professional Development Folder, otherwise known as the thing gathering dust on a shelf that you can never find and the thing you'll regret not keeping up to date when the new revalidation procedures begin to bite.

GP specialists can undertake a wide range of extended surgical skills as long as the training is

☢ Some of you older readers may remember the time-honoured phrase 'See one, do one, teach one'. Sorry, it's been consigned to history and should be used only during reminiscences after a few drinks on a Friday evening!

adequate and the necessary approvals are in place. Usually PCTs will support these activities as long as it is satisfied that it represents better value than carting the patient off to the hospital.

The procedures that were listed in the 1992 NHS Regulations are now included in the list of enhanced services.

You still need to be adequately skilled for these:

Incisions	Abscesses, cysts, thrombosed piles
Excisions	Cysts, lipomata, warts, ganglions, toenail removal, naevi, papillomata, dermatofibromata and similar lesions, plus skin lesions for biopsy
Aspirations	Joints, cysts, bursae, hydrocoeles
Injections	Intra-articular, peri-articular, varicose veins, haemorrhoids
Curettage, cautery and cryotherapy	Warts, verrucae and other skin lesions such as molluscum contagiosum
Other procedures	Removal of foreign bodies, nasal cautery

There are a few other things you need to think about:

THE FACILITIES

- Is the room of an adequate size – there are no regulations but $14\,m^2$ is generally considered reasonable.
- Is it well lit?
- Does it afford adequate privacy?
- Are there suitable operating lights?
- Are dressing trolleys available?
- Is there a suitable instrument cupboard?
- Are there sharps bins?
- Is there a general (non-clinical) waste bin?
- Are washing and hand-drying facilities adequate?
- Do you dispose of sharps in an approved manner?
- Is there a recovery facility for the patient who might feel unwell after undergoing a procedure?

WHAT ABOUT THE ASSISTANT?

The assistant, who should have adequate training, will be essential for:

- holding instruments
- assisting with sutures and ligatures
- adjusting lighting
- preparing instruments and dressing packs
- ensuring specimens are labelled and packed for despatch.

EQUIPMENT

- Is it appropriate for the task for which it is to be used?
- Is it fully serviceable?
- Is it free of rust?
- Does it meet the appropriate British Standard?
- Is it cleaned and fully sterilised (by autoclave) before use or is it disposable and single use?
- Is the sterilisation equipment regularly maintained (and is all the documentation available for inspection if necessary)?

And, by the way:

- Are instruments and packs sterilised using a local Central Sterile Supplies Department?
- Is any equipment requiring regular checking inspected to an agreed timetable and the results recorded?
- Is the resuscitation equipment regularly checked and the inspections recorded?
- Is a resuscitation poster displayed on the wall and available to everyone?

> **☢ Hazard warning**
>
> In a case of vasectomy a written consent must be obtained covering the following points:
>
> - The operation should be regarded as permanent.
> - It should not be regarded as successful until two negative sperm counts have been obtained and the patient informed in writing.
> - Advice that alternative contraception should be used in the meantime.
> - That there is a risk of late reversal if the tubes spontaneously rejoin.
>
> Where possible, have the consent signed by the patient and the partner. If the partner declines to sign, record the reason why.

ASSESSMENT, INFORMATION AND CONSENT

- Is the lesion suitable for surgery in the practice or is it better done in the hospital? (☢ Doctors frequently get into trouble when they take on procedures that are too complex for them.)
- Are there particular circumstances that might make the surgery unwise, e.g. excessive scarring or risk of malignancy?
- Does the patient have an unsuitable medical history, e.g. compromised circulation or complex medication?
- Do you ensure that you examine the patient and the lesion to be treated in advance of undertaking the procedure?
- Do you give the patient a full explanation of what is to happen?
- Do you give advice to the patient on any after-effects, the journey home, time off work and timing of suture removal?
- Do you have an 'Operator's Book' to record details of the procedure, however minor? You should record the date of procedure, nature of the procedure, type of anaesthetic used, name of operator and assistant and any complications noted during the procedure.
- Do you put full details of the procedure in the patient's notes?
- Do you have patient leaflets explaining post-operative care and effects such as pain or bleeding?
- Is the patient's consent obtained and recorded?

ANAESTHESIA

Modern anaesthesia has revolutionised surgical practice and made a great deal more minor surgery possible. The most popular is lignocaine, used either plain or with adrenaline and either infiltrated into the field of operation or used to block a particular nerve.

✎ The maximum safe dose of lignocaine for the proverbial 70 kg adult is 200 mg (equivalent to 20 ml of 1% lignocaine). If adrenaline is included in the anaesthetic the maximum dose increases to 500 mg (equivalent to 50 ml of 1% adrenaline).

Local anaesthetic may be supplemented by intravenous diazepam to produce an analgesic effect. The patient remains conscious but has no recollection of the procedure afterwards.

Diazepam may cause hallucinations, including those of a sexual nature – so the operator should ensure that he is chaperoned (or assisted) during the procedure.

What about general anaesthesia? Forget it! It is inappropriate outside hospital and you will probably not be able to get professional indemnity insurance to do it.

TECHNIQUE

✍ Another checklist for you to make a note of!

- Where appropriate, mark the lesion with an indelible marker.
- Ensure, where possible, incisions follow natural skin creases or Langer's lines.
- Be sure to avoid any superficial nerves or blood vessels.
- Scrub up and clean the operation site with antiseptic. It is wise to use coloured antiseptic visible to the patient.
- Ensure incisions are elliptical to prevent 'dog ears' during closure.
- Consider cosmetics (how the treatment will look, in the months and years to come) – they are a potent cause of complaint no matter how successful the actual surgery.
- Suture carefully with appropriate material and ensure they are not left in situ for longer than necessary.

HISTOPATHOLOGY

Many surgical procedures undertaken at the practice will involve the removal of a skin lesion. It is the surgeon's responsibility to:

- ensure that the sample is placed in a suitable transport medium (supplied by the histology department)
- ensure that the specimen is correctly, clearly and indelibly labelled
- ensure that the result is returned
- ensure that you act on the result if further treatment or referral is required
- record the sending of the specimen and the return of the result in the operation book

☢ Ensure that the patient is notified of the result. In the case of a normal result, it is good practice to do so. If there is an abnormality it will be considered negligent not to do so.

☹ WHAT HAPPENS WHEN IT ALL GOES WRONG?

Remember Murphy's Law – if it can go wrong it will. It may well be that the doctor was fully trained, followed the accepted guidelines, used a standard technique and properly managed the procedure in a suitable environment. Yet something went wrong!

The doctor's approach will certainly provide a defence but, if complications arise, there are some other things that must be done:

- Inform the patient of the complication without embellishment.
- Apologise for the unforeseen event.
- Fully record and examine the complication or damage before deciding whether to attempt a repair or refer it to a specialist colleague.
- Ensure that the complication is treated and rectified as soon as possible.

DEALING WITH DIFFICULT PATIENTS

In the vast majority of cases patients' behaviour and attitudes pose no problems, but every practitioner has patients who can be described as **difficult**. Although generally small in number, they take up a disproportionate amount of time.

They may cause problems in a number of ways:

- They may be rude or aggressive to the GP.
- They may be consistently aggressive and demanding to the receptionist but always perfectly charming when they see the GP.
- Rarely they may cause actual physical violence.
- They may waste practice time by, for example, failing to turn up for arranged appointments, etc.
- They may simply have the sort of personality that clashes with the GP.

Not every difficult patient presents a problem that is purely vexatious. Remember:

- The patient may simply be responding to rude, aggressive or unhelpful practice staff.
- Pain may impair their ability to behave in a socially acceptable manner.
- They may have a mental disorder which modifies their ability to be courteous.
- They may feel aggrieved about previous care (if it failed to bring relief of symptoms).
- The patient may be having a bad day(!).
- The patient may feel offended or fobbed off by the GP or staff.
- The patient may simply be rude or ignorant.

MISSED APPOINTMENTS

Practice efficiency can be disrupted when patients miss appointments without prior notification.

If a patient misses an appointment it may be appropriate to write to the person, but before doing so it is important to:

- establish that the patient did not cancel the appointment – patients are really annoyed if wrongly accused of failing to attend
- decide whether it is better to forget it or mention it at a future appointment.

Remember that letters are often seen by people other than the person to whom it was addressed. Ensure the tone strikes the right balance of concern whilst explaining the problems that failure to attend actually causes.

DIFFICULT PATIENTS

Every problem patient presents a unique dilemma for the practice. Management depends on the nature, frequency and seriousness of the problems that occur. You may consider:

- ignoring a single episode of inappropriate behaviour
- writing to the patient about it
- speaking to the patient about it or asking the senior partner to do so
- in serious cases arranging for the patient to be removed from the practice list.

Each of these approaches has advantages and disadvantages. Patients often refuse to accept that their behaviour was in any way difficult, particularly if they did not think that they actually were!

1 **Ignore a single incident:** It may be expedient to ignore one incident, especially if the patient is

Rebuking a difficult patient and particularly removing them from the list could lead to retaliation in the form of a complaint either to the PCT or to the GMC. If removal could be deemed 'unreasonable', it might be investigated by the Health Ombudsman.

known and the action is out of character. We all have bad days! It is advisable to:

- note the date and time of the incident and an account of what happened
- record actual comments if possible
- indicate which members of the practice were present when the incident occurred
- make a note of why the event caused distress
- decide at subsequent appointments whether to mention it to the patient or simply forget it
- if the patient makes an apology for an outburst, note it in the record. Sadly, apologising is no guarantee that it will not happen again.

2 **Write to the patient:** It may be appropriate to explain to the patient why their behaviour was not acceptable to you or the practice (e.g. racist comments). You may suggest that the patient comes to meet you to discuss the behaviour and how to manage it in future.

If the letter concerns inappropriate advances to partners or practice staff:

- It should follow a meeting of all GPs, to ensure that the patient is seen by another GP, normally of the same sex as the patient in future.

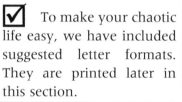

- The letter should be written by the senior partner and should advise the patient that he or she must be seen by another (named) doctor in future, and that the inappropriate attention is neither appreciated nor reciprocated.

  ☑ To make your chaotic life easy, we have included suggested letter formats. They are printed later in this section.

- If the GP is in a single-handed practice, the letter should state clearly that such advances are neither appreciated nor reciprocated and that the patient cannot remain on the list.

If the letter is to notify the patient that a particular type of behaviour is unacceptable:

- It should refer to the date and time of the incident in question.
- The letter should indicate who was present when the incident took place.
- It should clearly outline the alleged behaviour that is causing concern to the practice.
- It should make clear that any repetition of the behaviour would be regarded as unacceptable and might lead to removal from the list.
- It should give the patient the opportunity to come to see either the GP

or the practice manager to put his or her side of the story if the account in the letter is disputed.

If the letter is to invite the patient to come to the surgery to discuss his or her behaviour:

- Advise the patient of the alleged unacceptable events that have occurred.
- Inform the patient that the senior partner or the practice manager would like to see him or her to discuss the matter and to listen to the patient's account of events.

3 **Meeting the patient for conciliation:** The main purpose of such a meeting is to resolve any conflict that has arisen between the patient and the practice so that the professional relationship can return to its normal footing. At the meeting it would be wise to consider the following points:

- The meeting should not be too formal but should not appear casual.
- The individual leading the procedure for the practice should be accompanied. For example, if the senior partner, he or she should be accompanied by the practice manager.
- Practice representatives should try to enter into these discussions with an open mind.
- GPs and staff at the meeting should give the patient a clear outline of their concerns and explain why it was unacceptable.
- The patient should then have the opportunity to confirm or refute the practice's assessment of events.
- Once the events are agreed the patient and the practice should agree to rectify any identified areas of unacceptable behaviour or practice activity.

4 **Removing patients:** Under the new GMS arrangements a practice (and for all practical purposes that means a GP), with good reason, may have a patient removed from their list by notifying the PCT.

> ☑ Removal takes place on the day the patient is accepted by, or assigned to, another doctor, or eight days after the PCT receives the notification.

If a patient is involved in a violent act the doctor can arrange for an immediate removal by notifying the PCT in writing (by facsimile confirmed by hard copy) and by reporting the incident to the police and obtaining a crime number.

Removal of a patient should always be a last resort and the days when a GP could remove someone without offering a reason are now effectively gone.

Here's what the collective wisdom of the GMC has said on the matter:

'Rarely there may be circumstances in which you find it necessary to end your professional relationship with the patient. You must be satisfied your decision is fair . . . you must be prepared to justify your decision if called upon to do so

In such cases you should tell the patient why you have made this decision. You must also take steps to ensure that arrangements are made quickly for the continuing care of the patient.'

Removing any patient from the practice list should be carefully handled.

Warnings should be issued if necessary and counselling for the patient may be appropriate before invoking the removal process.

Removal may occur for a host of reasons. Assuming that the patient is over-demanding, offensive or unreliable, a suitable process for handling the situation might be as follows:

☢ The Health Service Commissioner for England and Wales (the Ombudsman) has shown himself prepared to 'name and shame' any GP removing a patient from the list when investigation fails to demonstrate a good reason and the doctor has refused to apologise.

- Document incidents where the patient's behaviour is unacceptable and raise them with the patient at the first opportunity.
- Invite the patient to attend the surgery to discuss his or her future relationship with the doctor and the practice.
- Discuss the matter in the presence of the practice manager who should take notes. A copy of the notes and agreed changes should be given to the patient and another kept in the medical record.
- Any further deviations from the agreement should be recorded in the medical record.
- If the unacceptable behaviour continues the doctor should write a letter to the patient explaining why it is no longer possible to provide care and outlining the areas where the ability to do so has broken down.

SUGGESTED DRAFT LETTERS

Warning about future behaviour

Dear *[insert name]*

I understand from *[person's name]* that an incident occurred at the practice on *[date]* at *[time]*. It involved *[describe the incident]*.

I would be grateful if you could let me know in writing if my understanding of the sequence of events is in any way incorrect.

The practice does its best to provide the highest standards of care for the patients, but we require support and co-operation. We cannot allow incidents of this sort to pass unnoticed and I must inform you that if there is any repetition of this behaviour it may not be possible to provide any further treatment.

The practice is here to assist you and I hope that we can work together in future to meet your expectations of us and our expectations of you.

Yours sincerely,

Dr A Practitioner

Taking no action

Dear *[insert name]*

I understand that an incident occurred at the practice on *[date]* at *[time]*.

I have investigated the matter *[and noted your comments]*. I have accordingly decided to take no action on this occasion.

However, I must point out that successful care depends on mutual co-operation and I hope we shall be able to enjoy a better professional relationship in future.

We are here to help you but we cannot accede to unreasonable demands.

Yours sincerely,

Dr A Practitioner

Missed appointment

Dear *[insert name]*

It has come to my notice that you failed to attend your appointment on *[date]*.

Our objective is to provide the best service we can for our patients but we do need patients' co-operation to do this.

Wasting appointments impedes our ability to see all the patients who need consultations.

Consequently, if you need to cancel an appointment again we would be grateful if you could notify reception in good time so that it can be given to another patient.

Yours sincerely,

Dr A Practitioner

Many missed appointments

Dear *[insert name]*

You have failed to attend for *[number]* appointments over the past *[number]* weeks.

Repeated failure to keep your appointments not only causes inconvenience but also denies other patients the opportunity to see the doctor.

Please be advised that if you fail to attend any further appointments without good reason we may need to ask the Primary Care Trust to remove your name from our list of patients.

Yours sincerely,

Dr A Practitioner

Patient removal from the practice list

Dear *[insert name]*

[As you are aware] the practice has had concerns about certain aspects of your *[conduct/behaviour]* for a considerable period of time.

I advised you about these concerns *[by letter/at our consultation on day-month-year]* and it was agreed *[in the notes of that meeting which were sent/given to you]* that you would take steps to resolve the difficulty *[I enclose a further copy of these notes for your information]*.

There has been no improvement and further incidents have occurred *[give a description of the events since the letter/meeting]*. The point has now been reached where these continued problems have so seriously damaged the relationship of mutual trust and co-operation that existed between us that I no longer feel able to provide you with care to the standard that I feel is appropriate.

I am therefore taking steps to have your name removed from the practice's list of patients.

Please make arrangements to register with another doctor. If you have any difficulty in doing so, please contact *[name]* PCT at *[address]* and a member of the staff will arrange for you to be allocated to a new GP.

[Optional] I shall delay sending the notification to the PCT for three days from the date of this letter. If you feel that it will be possible to resolve the issues which I have outlined and normalise our professional relationship, please contact the practice manager on *[telephone number]* and arrange an appointment for us to meet.

I am very disappointed that it has proved to be impossible for us to maintain a satisfactory professional relationship. May I offer you every good wish for the future.

Yours sincerely,

Dr A Practitioner

There is always a difficult judgement to be made about deciding to take action or ignoring unacceptable episodes and the decision will depend on an array of circumstances.

Sometimes it is not appropriate to stir up a hornet's nest but on other occasions ignoring behaviour that is unacceptable may simply result in it being repeated at a later appointment.

☺ The last word on the subject . . . contact your defence organisation insurance medicolegal adviser and discuss the problem before taking action. An independent view may help to resolve or manage the problem.

OK, several words but they are very wise!

CONSENT

Patients have a right to information about their condition. The amount of information with which they are provided will vary according to the nature, severity and complexity of that condition.

Any GP who treats a patient without their valid consent may face:

> ☢ In the United Kingdom any competent adult has the right to give or withhold consent to any examination, investigation or treatment.

- a criminal action for 'battery' (in England and Wales) or assault (in Scotland)
- a civil action for negligence.

In England and Wales 'battery' is the injuring or even touching of another person deliberately without his or her consent. Therefore battery can lead to a criminal prosecution or a civil claim for compensation. However, a GP is most unlikely to be accused of criminal battery because it requires ill-intent, which would be very difficult to demonstrate.

There are two types of consent:

- implied
- expressed, which may be verbal or written.

Many people believe that a written consent has greater validity than a verbal consent. Under some circumstances this could be true. The signed consent form does indicate that something connected with the consent occurred and the patient signed a

> ☢ Take great care with implied consent and accept it only for the most basic of procedures. For example, if a patient opens his mouth, there is an implied consent that you may examine his throat visually. To do more requires a more formalised consent, to explain what you intend to do and why.

piece of paper agreeing to something. However, most consent forms do not detail the areas of the procedure that were discussed and for that reason, well-written notes explaining the issues considered and written contemporaneously are just as valid.

Where a verbal consent is obtained, you must make a good clear, contemporaneous record of it.

> **⊕ Remember**
> No notes, no defence.

> ☑ The GMC provides a comprehensive booklet about consent and how the GP should approach the issues in a range of circumstances. GPs are strongly advised to comply with the regulatory body requirements. Failure to do so will be extremely difficult to defend in the event of a complaint.
>
> GMC documentation concerning standards and behaviour is regarded as the authoritative guidance to comply with. Using the *Bolam* test, the likelihood is that a reasonable body of peers would meet the requirement and obtain written consent.

As with all questions about the conduct of, or treatment provided by a GP, an allegation may not emerge until months or even years after the event.

To be asked to recall an incident that happened years previously and to try to establish whether you obtained some sort of valid consent would be impossible without a suitable note in the record.

It is helpful to develop a habit of always writing a note stating that the risks, benefits and alternatives have been discussed. It takes a few seconds and may protect you from days, weeks or years of heartache if a patient accuses you of treatment without consent.

Consent must be **valid**. Sometimes consent is described as informed. In our view, 'informed' is an inappropriate term (although it is popular in the United States) because, we would argue, consent cannot be uninformed.

In other words, a patient cannot consent to something that he or she does not understand.

However, to be **valid** requires the GP to tell the patient enough information to enable them to make an informed decision. The amount of information will vary according to the nature and complexity of the condition requiring treatment or investigation, but it may well include:

• details of diagnosis and prognosis
• uncertainties about diagnosis
• options for treatment
• the purpose of the procedure(s) and the possible consequences

- the benefits and disadvantages
- possible side-effects
- the option of not treating the patient and the consequences.

> ☑ It must be made clear to patients that they may change their mind at any stage during a course of treatment.

One of the great difficulties for clinicians of all sorts is that, once they have convinced themselves that a particular course of treatment will provide benefit for the patient, it is very difficult not to advocate it to the exclusion of any other possible alternatives.

> ☢ **Remember**
> Consent is a process, not an event!

It does not matter how much better you believe your treatment will make the patient. **If the patient does not consent to it, you must not do it.** Any competent adult can refuse any treatment at any time and as a professional clinician, you must respect it. In some circumstances patients refuse treatment that will prolong or

> 💡 **Think about this clinical point:**
> A well-known example of potential 'serious' harm is where a patient develops unilateral temporary blindness and where multiple sclerosis is the suspected diagnosis. Following resolution there are no further symptoms (40% of patients never develop other features of the disease). It may be considered capable of causing **serious harm** at a later stage to tell an asymptomatic patient that they might have multiple sclerosis.

preserve life. Provided they are competent they have a perfect right to do so.

Some patients are very inquisitive and ask many questions about proposed care. The GP really has an obligation to answer all the questions as honestly, fully and objectively as possible.

Information can only be withheld from a patient if you believe that the disclosure would cause the patient **serious** harm. Like many things in healthcare, the term 'serious' in not, in this context, defined and is a matter for the clinician's judgement.

However, 'serious' should not be taken to mean that the patient would become upset. It implies a much more profound state of distress than that. In all aspects of conduct, the GP should keep in mind that he or she should act in a way that is reasonable and defensible. If a complaint about his or her conduct arises subsequently, the onus will be to explain and justify the actions. In the context of consent the GP will need to explain what information was provided and demonstrate that it was adequate.

Wherever possible the GP should explain personally to the patient about proposed treatment and obtain the consent himself. The GP has the responsibility to ensure that the consent process is completed satisfactorily. However, the process may be delegated to a suitably trained and qualified colleague who has sufficient knowledge of the procedure, risks and alternatives.

 Hazard warning
When competence is in doubt; write copious notes. You may have to depend on them if questions arise later.

Competence is the central issue in deciding whether a patient can give consent to a procedure. Competence should be assessed by the clinician managing the case. For a patient to be regarded as competent he or she should meet the following criteria:

- understand the nature and purpose of the treatment
- understand the benefits, risks and alternatives to the treatment
- understand the consequences of refusing treatment

If there is any doubt a GP should refer for a psychiatric or psycho-geriatric review to assess competence.

- be able to retain the information long enough to make a reasoned decision
- be able to make a free choice (i.e. not act under duress).

There may be cases where the GP is unable to decide whether a patient is competent. In such situations a clearer picture may be obtained by seeking the views of friends, relatives or carers (see below). It is sometimes a difficult decision and the GP should be careful to document the stages in reaching the conclusion.

A patient may be incompetent, that is, unable to meet the criteria for competence. **In the United Kingdom no one can give consent for another adult.**

The GP must **act in the patient's best interests.** In order to make the decision the GP should:

- Try to ascertain the past wishes of the patient.
- Try to encourage the person to participate in the decision if possible. In some (particularly elderly) patients there may be a tendency for them to drift in and out of competence. It may require time to establish their true wishes.
- Consult with friends, relatives and carers and any other appropriate people.

- Consider the options for treatment with a view to providing the therapy that will achieve the desired result with the minimum of intervention.

CHILDREN

However difficult the process of consent may appear to be for adults, it is much more complicated in some circumstances involving children.

Competent children aged 16 or over

Such children may be regarded as adults for the purposes of consent. The position is enshrined in the Family Law Reform Act (1969) Section 8.1. **In case you don't have a copy to hand, here's what it says:**

> 'The consent of a minor who has attained the age of sixteen years to any surgical, medical or dental treatment which, in the absence of consent, would constitute a trespass to his person, shall be as effective as it would be if he were of full age; and where the minor has by virtue of this section given an effective consent to any treatment it shall not be necessary to obtain any consent for it from his parent or guardian.'

It is important to note that this statute is confined to consent, **not to refusal**, where parents retain residual rights to overrule the refusal of a child to accept a procedure.

Of course, the reality of the situation is that when confronted by a burly 17-year-old refusing to have treatment and a mother saying she wants it done, only a foolhardy GP would wade in and try to do it.

In these circumstances negotiation is the key and it is very unwise to try to force any treatment of any sort on a child who is adamant that they don't want it.

Incompetent children aged 16 or over

With respect to consent, these children are covered by common law. Parents can consent for children who are incompetent when aged 16 or 17.

Children aged under 16

A child below the age of 16 has the right to make his or her own decision upon demonstrating sufficient maturity to understand the nature of the matter requiring decision.

The Gillick case

This now-famous case concerned the prescription of oral contraceptives to the daughters of Mrs Victoria Gillick without her involvement or consent. She subsequently took legal action against the health authority and the prescribing doctor (*Gillick* v *West Norfolk and Wisbech Area Health Authority et al. [1986]*). In a case that attracted considerable publicity and discussion, the judge decided in favour of the health authority and the doctor and pronounced that the assessment of children below the age of 16 is a matter for the doctor and his clinical judgement, subject to:

- the child understanding the issues surrounding the prescription and use of the drug (i.e. competence)
- the doctor being unable to convince the child that she should inform her parents
- a judgement that the child was likely to have sexual intercourse in any event
- a concern that, without appropriate contraceptive advice, the child's physical or mental health may suffer
- her best interests being served.

Clearly this judgement related only to a narrow element of medical care but the concept has been rolled out across the whole of healthcare. Therefore if confronted by a child below the age of 16 he or she may be treated by the GP if satisfied that the child is competent.

It is important to note that, as with children below 18, the ruling is confined to consent and not to refusal. More about 'refusal' follows, below.

In essence 'Gillick competence' recognises the right of self-determination of young persons. It acknowledges that parental rights over children are dwindling and that they can be overridden. In essence the rights of parents are now only residual and are wholly extinguished at the age of majority.

In Scotland, the issue of children under 16 consenting to treatment is detailed in the Age of Legal Capacity (Scotland) Act 1991. The Act says:

> 'A person under the age of sixteen years shall have the legal capacity to consent on his own behalf to any surgical, medical or dental procedure or treatment where, in the opinion of a qualified medical practitioner attending him, he is capable of understanding the nature and possible consequences of the procedure or treatment.'

Refusal of treatment by children up to the age of 18 is treated differently. Parents can override a refusal (though not consent). Refusal (and consent) can also be overridden by a court if it is in the patient's best interests.

For the GP a child refusing treatment clearly raises issues beyond

> From a legal point of view there is asymmetry between consent and refusal because a child's consent is enabling (allows the treatment to proceed) but refusal is **not** disabling (because that consent can be exercised by another).

those of obtaining consent from a parent. A young person determined not to accept treatment is effectively untreatable and it is usually very unwise to try to force treatment on an unwilling child.

In certain medical circumstances a degree of coercion may be useful where a particular medical treatment is essential and parental consent is obtained, but in general practice when negotiation fails it is often better to accept that treatment will not be possible and to rearrange an appointment.

Consider these cases:

> **☺ Exercise**
>
> A patient with a painful knee sits down in your consulting room, removes her stocking and turns the knee towards you.
>
> Do you need her consent to **look** at the knee?

> **☺ Exercise**
>
> Halfway through a course of treatment, the patient decided that he did not want any more treatment. You remonstrate with him saying that the course is nearly finished and he should really complete it.
>
> The man insists that he wants to stop.
>
> Should you assist him to find alternative treatment or insist that he finishes the treatment that you regard as best?

> **Take break!** You have our consent, after reading this far – you need one!

CONFIDENTIALITY

We all expect our most personal information to be kept secret. In a world where communications are becoming easier and more information is available to more people, it is getting increasingly difficult.

However, being a GP brings with it certain privileges and one of them is that you can ask patients all sorts of personal questions of a confidential nature. What is more, it is reasonable to expect answers and if the answers are not forthcoming, you have the right to refuse to undertake the treatment.

However, the privilege of being able to access confidential information brings with it an ethical obligation to maintain that information confidential.

Confidentiality is a central tenet of the relationship between patient and GP, as with all other healthcare professionals. It has been a vital part of the code of medical ethics throughout history.

The Hippocratic Oath states:

> 'All that may come into my knowledge in the exercise of my profession or in daily commerce with men, which ought not to be spread abroad, I will keep secret and will never reveal.'

The Oath was modified by the **Declaration of Geneva** to read:

> 'I will respect the secrets which are confided in me, even after the patient has died.'

Of course you don't need the pronouncement of a white-haired bearded old Greek, or a bunch of Swiss gnomes, to know that everything you learn in the privacy of the consulting room should be kept confidential.

> ☢ If in doubt, keep it confidential and seek advice from insurance company advisers.

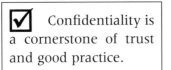 Confidentiality is a cornerstone of trust and good practice.

Confidentiality will almost always be **absolute**. It is a key requirement of good practice. If GPs did not keep confidential what they learn during the course of consultations, they would not attract the confidence of patients.

Patients would not want to confide information for fear that it might be passed on to others. Release of inappropriate information could lead to stigmatisation and discrimination.

Indeed, if patients withhold information from their healthcare professionals, their treatment might be compromised, particularly if a decision on management were to be made in the absence of key relevant detail.

Worse still, a patient in need of treatment might decide not to attend a GP altogether if he or she felt that there was a significant risk of breach of confidence.

☑ Every GP should eat, sleep and read GMC Guidance every day.
    Yeah, right! Well, at least we've said it.

The General Medical Council takes a firm view on confidentiality. It produces a comprehensive booklet on confidentiality that outlines the ethical duties of a GP. Every GP should know the document like the back of their hand.

Of course, during the course of a consultation there will be a barrage of information often being made available. Is it all confidential?

☺ Exercise
Here are some other conundrums:
    If a schoolteacher asks whether a child has come for treatment at a certain time, should you confirm it?
    If the police ask you about a patient attendance, should you tell them?
    Should a wife know that her husband is HIV positive?

Is it reasonable, for instance, to tell a husband, if he rings the surgery, that his wife has come in for medical treatment or is such information confidential?

Aside from any ethical or legal considerations, it is important to consider the release of information from the patient's perspective. If it were your information, would you want it to be released to other people without your consent? This is a highly emotional question. Fortunately the law helps us with many of the answers for the question: what constitutes confidential information?

Several court cases have established a **legal duty of confidence**. Some of the elements are really back-to-front and describe those characteristics of information that are what is called a 'breach'. The language is pretty clunky! Here they are:

- Information must have the necessary quality of confidence.
- Information must be disclosed in circumstances implying an obligation of confidence.

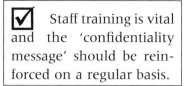 Staff training is vital and the 'confidentiality message' should be reinforced on a regular basis.

- Unauthorised disclosure would cause harm to the confider.
- The disclosure itself would have the potential to harm the patient in the future.

In plain English? In essence these criteria make clear that information provided in the privacy of a consulting room must be regarded as confidential. The consulting room environment certainly implies an obligation of confidence and any disclosure of information would be a breach of the obligation, whether or not any actual harm had occurred.

It is important to remember that the duty of confidentiality extends to the members of the practice team.

A GP has a legal responsibility for members of the team. Do you

☢ Consider a young woman patient, with her mother in attendance, consulting about (say) a painful shoulder. It would be wholly inappropriate to release information, for example, about her medical history.

If it became necessary, for instance, to confirm that the woman was still taking an oral contraceptive pill, it would be necessary to find a way of asking the question at a time when the patient was alone. Furthermore, GPs should be very careful about answering even apparently innocent questions posed by relatives during the course of a consultation.

know what your receptionist is saying when you are not there? Breaches of confidentiality by staff are a serious disciplinary matter for the practice.

Sometimes patients bring with them family members or friends to act as a chaperone or merely to provide some moral support. GPs should be very cautious about what is said in the presence of others.

Of course, over time, professional relationships develop between practitioners and their clients. Sometimes it is very difficult to keep confidential any information concerning third parties about which you may be asked.

Rather than a brusque 'I cannot tell you', developing a stock phrase such as 'Unfortunately my professional code prevents me from telling you' sounds less like telling them to mind their own business.

KIDS: AGAIN

☑ In circumstances where data is requested GPs should look carefully at the information provided.

If they have any doubt that it is appropriate to supply all the information, they should discuss the matter with the patient and get a signed consent confirming what is to be released.

If the patient asks for information to be withheld from a solicitor or insurer for instance the GP should make clear in supplying the data that some information was being withheld at the request of the patient. Such a situation might arise for example where a solicitor is reviewing an accident six months earlier but asks for records dating back 20 years. The GP may well feel it is wise to enquire of the patient whether he or she wishes to part with all the information to the solicitor.

As with consent, children provide a special problem for the GP. The age at which a child will be able to consent to treatment, i.e. becomes competent to make the decision, will vary according to the degree of judgement and maturity that the child can apply.

In reality the GP should be able to discuss confidential medical matters with the parents of any child who is not considered competent to make his or her own decisions. Once they are competent, at whatever age, they acquire the right to confidentiality enshrined in the *Gillick* judgement.

The same situation applies with patients who have mental health problems, or learning disabilities. If the patient has, in the opinion of the clinician, a sufficient level of understanding then they have the right to consent and therefore the right to retain control over disclosure of their own records.

JUSTIFIED DISCLOSURE

There are certain circumstances where disclosure of patient information may be considered justified. **Justified disclosure** is relatively rare and in the vast majority of circumstances absolute confidentiality should apply. Clearly the information imparted to the GP belongs to the patient and the patient normally has the right to choose when and to whom he or she wishes to impart that information.

In some circumstances the patient will consent to the GP releasing information that would normally be regarded as confidential to third parties.

Such third parties might include:

> ☑ If parting with notes to an insurance company or solicitor, make sure that there is a recently signed consent covering the whole release.

- other healthcare professionals to whom the patient is referred or who might be involved in providing care for the patient
- insurance companies seeking information relating to claims for injuries or other matters where the GP is in possession of that information
- solicitors acting for the patient or for others.

Are there circumstances where disclosure may be justified **without** the patient's consent?

Yes, here they are:

- **Where there is a legal or statutory requirement:**

  > ☑ Never part with records without taking a photocopy first.

  - certain Acts of Parliament, for example if a patient is suspected of being a terrorist
  - serious injury or dangerous occurrence.
- **When ordered to do so by a court:** If the GP receives a court order instructing him to release his records, then he must comply with the order. However, if the request comes from a court official or a lawyer without a court order, there is no requirement to release the records unless there is another ground. If the records are required by a coroner's officer (police officer) then the GP should comply.
- **Where there are medical grounds:** Such a circumstance might be to the relative of a patient with a terminal illness in order to assist the relative in providing the necessary care.

> ☢ There are two important things to remember when disclosing confidential information.
> 1 Write hugely comprehensive notes. If there is a to-do about the release later, those friendly people at the GMC may ask you to explain and justify your reasons for releasing the information. Woe betide you if you can't remember why you did it!
> 2 Only release information to the appropriate authority. Breaching confidentiality does not mean that you can tell the world and his wife.

- **In the public interest:** Such a situation may occur where there is a substantial risk that failure to disclose information may result in the patient suffering harm or death or someone else suffering harm or death. The GP has to decide whether the duty of care to an individual or to society overrides the duty of confidentiality to the patient.

If you are confronted with a request to breach the confidentiality of a patient there are a number of questions that you should ask in trying to assess whether such a breach would be reasonable:

- What information does the enquirer want to know? Be clear about what they want.
- Why do they want to know it? Is there some other way that they can find out the information without the need for you to breach confidentiality?
- By what authority do they seek it? Do they have a court order or some other authority that gives them a right to the information?
- What grounds can justify the release of the information? A GP placed in a situation like this has to recognise that, whatever decision is made, he or she will be very unpopular with someone. In situations where a release is required the GP should:
  - have a period of quiet reflection to assist him in deciding what to do
  - contact the medico-legal adviser at the medical defence insurer and discuss the matter.

Remember that patient autonomy is the central feature of confidentiality and is paramount. It is only in a very small number of cases that there is a justification for the release of any confidential information.

> ☺ The information belongs to the patient and the patient will normally always have the right to decide when and if the information is released to someone else.

Breaching confidentiality will cause patients to lose trust and confidence in the profession resulting in inadequate information or failures to attend for treatment.

THE POLICE

Because of the confusion that may surround enquiries by police, it is worth taking a specific look.

The police do not have a blanket permission to obtain information about patients. There are no hard and fast rules about releasing information – so a GP must make a judgement.

However, if that judgement is called into question at a later stage he or she may be required to explain and justify his or her actions to the GMC if a patient lodges a complaint about breach of confidentiality.

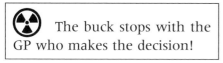 The buck stops with the GP who makes the decision!

The following points may be helpful as general guidance if the police come knocking on the door:

1 Remember that apparently innocent information like times of appointments or indeed even whether an individual is a patient may, under some circumstances, constitute a breach of confidentiality.
2 If police turn up at a surgery **without a court order** requiring information about a patient they do not have an automatic right to obtain it. A police uniform does not constitute authority.
3 If they present a Court Order signed by a Circuit Judge instructing you to release specific information, you **must** comply with the order. Make sure that you keep a fair copy of all the notes with which you part.
4 If police, without a court order, seek information about an alleged crime, which is of a minor nature, you may not have any obligation to release it without court direction, especially if it is hearsay or from a third party.

Changes in the new GMS contract make it vital that the practice has an agreed protocol for dealing with the issue of release of information to the police. It may be agreed that only the practice principals can make the decision, or any GP, or the practice manager. In any event, decide what you're going to do, document it as an operational procedure and be prepare to justify it!

5 If police without a court order seek information concerning a serious crime you may feel it appropriate to release it. You should be satisfied that the information being provided by the police is of an adequate standard and justification for the release. It may be that failure to do so may result in another crime being committed, that serious harm may befall individuals or that failure to release the information may result in the suspect evading justice.

6 Reception and other staff should be instructed **never** to release information to the police without the authority of the GP except in very exceptional circumstances.

7 If you receive a request for the release of records, always make a detailed note of the request, including:
   • the nature of the information requested
   • the details of the police officer(s) seeking the information
   • your decision whether to release it or not
   • your reasons for making the judgement.

8 Don't be bounced into releasing information, especially if you do not believe it to be appropriate to do so. If you are unsure, discuss it with your medical defence insurer. Don't be intimidated by a tall police officer because he is in uniform and carries a truncheon in his pocket!

PATIENT RECORDS AND THE LAW

GPs keep records for their own access to assist them in planning and treating patients and to remind them of treatment previously provided. Less than 35 years ago patients were normally prohibited access to their records. However, successive Acts of Parliament have given patients full access and the practice should understand what the Acts are and how they should comply.

THE DATA PROTECTION ACT 1984

This was the original Act permitting access to patient information held on computer record. The Act was repealed when the subsequent 1998 Data Protection Act was enacted.

THE ACCESS TO HEALTH RECORDS ACT 1990

This Act applied to manual records held by the practice. It gave patients the right of access to those records made after 1 November 1991, although practitioners could release all records if they wished to do so.

There were certain exemptions which were essentially the same as those incorporated in the 1998 Data Protection Act (see below). The Access to Health Records Act was repealed, in respect of living patients, when the Data Protection Act 1998 came into force.

The important exception is for deceased patients, whose records should still be processed under the provisions of the 1990 Act (that is, right of access to records made after 1 November 1991, although a practitioner may release all records if he or she wishes to do so). The request for records must be 'properly received'. That means: from the next of kin, the executor of the will or anyone who can demonstrate a pecuniary interest in the will.

THE DATA PROTECTION ACT 1998

The Act came into force on 1 March 2000. It repealed the earlier Act of 1984 and its provisions apply only to living individuals. The Act includes all manual health records and all electronic records, whenever they were made.

The Act applies UK-wide.

The Act sets out eight data protection principles. They state that data shall:

> ☢ Data protection legislation has got all sorts of organisations, from the police to gas companies, into a tangle. It looks like a very good smokescreen to hide behind. It is not. Getting on top of the legislation and what it means is very important. Worth taking the time to wrap your head around it.

> ☺ Health records are defined as: any records containing information relating to the physical or mental health of the individual (patient). It may include pictures, diagrams, photographs and video recordings.

- be processed fairly and lawfully
- be obtained only for specified and lawful purposes
- be adequate, relevant and not excessive
- be accurate and kept up-to-date
- not be kept for longer than necessary
- be processed in accordance with the rights of the data subject
- be held secure
- not be transferred to a country outside the EEA without adequate safeguards.

Patients may have access to their records under Section 7 of the Act. The request must be made in writing. A standard access fee of £10 is payable for electronic records but a further fee of up to £50 may be charged for paper records.

It has been suggested that 33p per sheet may be a suitable charge for manual records.

The Act provides for the documents to be supplied within 40 days.

The Act requires for the release of **all** records but there are specific exemptions.

The data controller (you!) can exclude any information that breaches the confidentiality of a third party (who is not a health professional and who has not consented to the disclosure).

> **Hazard warning**
>
> When any documents are destroyed they must be incinerated or shredded with appropriate safeguards for confidentiality throughout the procedure.

Disclosure may also be withheld if its release is likely to 'cause serious harm to the physical or mental health or condition of the data subject (patient) or any other person'. Causing serious harm does not mean that the patient might not like the information much, or indeed may be upset by it. It must cause **serious** harm. This latter restriction is unlikely to be encountered by a practice GP except in very occasional mental health cases and a few serious or terminal illnesses.

A patient can ask for inaccuracies in their record to be corrected. If they are dissatisfied they may complain to the Data Protection Commissioner or apply to the court for a court order for compliance.

> Patients can now claim compensation for damage or distress caused by a breach of the Act.

The court could order a GP to rectify, block, erase or destroy inaccurate data or require that the record be supplemented with a statement setting out the true facts.

NOTIFICATION

The Act requires that a data controller (that's you!) must provide the Data Protection Commissioner with certain particulars, including the name and address, a description of the personal data being processed, the purpose for the processing and a description of the recipients.

Any GP receiving a request for notes under the Data Protection Act, especially if there is concern that the search might be in contemplation of a claim, should contact the medico-legal adviser at the insurer for advice and guidance. It's a minefield of complexity and it's time to get your money's worth and let the medico-legal insurer earn their corn.

THE ACCESS TO MEDICAL REPORTS ACT 1988

This Act applies to reports supplied for employment or insurance purposes by a practitioner who has been responsible for the clinical care of the individual. If a request for a report is made, the request must be accompanied by a valid signed consent from the patient concerned or the practitioner must seek suitable consent to provide the report. The patient must also be notified that the report has been sought and has the right to see the report before it is sent to the employer or insurer if he or she chooses to do so.

If the patient chooses to see the report, the employer or insurance company must notify the practitioner about this. If the patient does not arrange access (to see the report), the practice must wait at least 21 days before sending off the report.

If the patient sees the report, he or she may ask the GP to amend any part of the report that is considered to be inaccurate. The GP may either comply with the patient's wishes or append to the report a statement of the patient's view. The GP must have written permission from the patient before sending off the report.

☢ Patients who choose **not** to see the report should sign a statement to this effect. However, they may change their mind by writing to the GP concerned and may see the report for up to six months afterwards.

MEDICAL RECORDS

Everyone knows the jokes about doctors' handwriting. And it is not getting any better!

But, as Bob Dylan so famously sang, 'The Times They Are A Changin''. A much greater focus is being placed on record keeping and a high standard is now expected.

Many changes may impact on record keeping. Here are just a few of them:

- patients having greater involvement in choices associated with their own care
- increasing patient centred, rather than task oriented, notes
- patient access to their records
- clinical audit and governance
- the routine use of computerised records.

We should first understand what constitutes a record. Well, like Enid Blyton, the records should contain a famous five:

1 Identify the patient.
2 Support the diagnosis by having a clear history and examination.
3 Justify the treatment.
4 Document the course and results and evaluate the outcome.
5 Be prepared to change therapies where effectiveness has not been demonstrated.

☑ The only thing you need to remember is: If it wasn't documented it wasn't done. Got that! That's it, nothing else. Finito.

☢ Research shows that up to 40% of claims for medical negligence are indefensible because of documentation problems.

Make a note of that! Better still, write it down!

☑ **Tip**
There is nothing a mischievous barrister likes more than to ask a GP to read a completely illegible entry in the notes that may have been written years earlier. It is easy to look **very, very** stupid.

☺ Remember, the notes may be all you have if a complaint or a claim is made weeks, months or even years later.

It is also nice to have some positive comments. Not essential, but descriptions of positive improvements may well be valuable if everything goes pear-shaped later on.

GP records were notoriously difficult to read, but with the advent of computerisation they have become clearer, despite some rather creative spelling by some doctors.

If a claim is made against you, you can be sure that the patient will be able to describe every last aspect of the consultation and treatment down to the length of time of the appointment and the colour of your nail varnish.

☑ Improve legibility by using black, non-fading ink.

You, on the other hand, will **only** have your notes and if they do not state your case well enough then you are in the proverbial. Take a couple of extra minutes to ensure that you do not cut any corners on your record keeping.

Watch out for the common risks.

Here's the Top 10:

Problem	Solution
Identity of patient, especially if two with the same or similar names	Make sure that the notes have a name hazard sticker on them.
Ensure that key elements of the past medical history are recorded	A standard checklist may avoid the occasional aberration.
Avoid abbreviations that confuse, e.g. PID	Yes, we all know it's Prolapsed Inter-vertebral Disc and not Pelvic Inflammatory Disease, or is it? Be very careful with abbreviations. Either write out terms in full or, if you use abbreviations regularly, provide a key that shows what each one means.
Consent	If they agreed to a course of treatment verbally, make a note that they did so and when.
Continuity of records	Ensure accuracy and that they clearly indicate progress or deterioration in the condition.
Disparaging comments	**Never** use disparaging comments or rude abbreviations. Patients can now see their records and they will be infuriated.
Audit and research	With increasing requirements for CPD and appraisal, ensure that notes can be used to extract data if necessary.
Delay in writing records	Notes should be contemporaneous, that is written within 24 hours (certainly no more than 48 hours) after the consultation.
Protection	Make sure they protect you and the patient.
Security	Make sure they are secure, unavailable to unauthorised persons and protected from damp, infestation, etc. You never know when you might need them! Make sure all computer records are adequately backed-up (see later).
Exposure to allegations of improper conduct	Have a chaperone available (*see* Annex 1)

ABSENCE OF INFORMATION

Absence of information is of course the key problem with legible and otherwise acceptable records.

It is no good professing that your treatments for arthritis produced a complete cure when the patient alleges, in a claim, that she cannot do the shopping, carry the children or walk around for more than five minutes.

If your contemporaneous notes said that she could walk three miles without pain and had resumed her pole-dancing career, you will be in a much stronger position.

Judges (and other people) are still inclined to believe contemporaneous notes. They were, after all, written before there was any suggestion of a problem in most cases. It is difficult to lie in notes when you don't know how things may turn out in the future.

> Do not be tempted to leave spaces in notes so that you can fill them in later, if you need to beef up your records.
>
> It might have worked years ago. Today ink can be forensically dated – embarrassing if the claimant's lawyer finds a sentence in the middle of the notes that is three years younger than the rest! Bear in mind that computer wizards can reveal a time-lined audit trail buried in your PC.

ALTERATIONS

Never, never, never destroy, alter or rewrite a previous record under any circumstances whatsoever, however tempted you may be.

You are bound to be found out, either by the forensic tests (if the patient or the lawyer suspects that you changed notes in circumstances that they remember differently) or because you make statements that do not accord with the situation at the time. Patients may well ask for a copy of their notes and if you forget and make an 'amendment' it will irreparably damage your credibility if it comes to light – likely if the patient's copy is different to your 'original'. Just don't do it.

In the case of computerised records, any suspicion of adjusting records can be easily discovered by a computer

> **Don't risk making any 'adjustments'**
>
> . . . it destroys your integrity and your professionalism.
>
> If you only want to know porridge as a warming breakfast cereal, **never** change a record.

boffin who can look into the dark recesses of your hard disc (and discover a thing called an audit trail) and find out exactly when each part of any entry was made.

Biased notes

Biased notes should be avoided. Try to avoid phrases such as 'the patient is always complaining' or 'the patient is too demanding'. It may be absolutely true but in the wrong place (such as a court) it will put you in a bad light.

It is also worth remembering that emotive comments such as 'patient had a good week' tend not to be very helpful. Did the patient have no symptoms, can she walk twice as far, is her pain now more bearable or did she really have a good week when she met Brad Pitt for an exuberant fling? Having a 'good week' has a lot of different meanings. Be explicit.

Good quality notes

Good quality notes are what most GPs produce. Check yours against this checklist and be sure that they comply. Good notes equal less risk and less chance of meeting those nice friendly lawyers and judges at the court or at the GMC!

	Always do	Sometimes	Err . . .
Patient details			
Current complaints			
History of current complaints			
Past medical history			
Social history			
Examination and findings			
Treatment plan			
Patient consent			
Progress of treatment. Ensure date recorded each time			
Measures of improvement or deterioration			
Changes of treatment			
Patient consent			
Dispersal			
Referral to specialist/colleague/reason			
Discharge – advice given and date			
Instructions for return if required			

Some more thoughts about notes

How much should you write?

The glib answer is, of course, as much as you need to! Some GPs take the view that the records should record all the findings from the history and the examination. Others feel that they should be written on the basis of exception reporting.

Experts take the view that both approaches are acceptable and that the parameter for successful notes is not how long they are.

Pages of meaningless drivel are valueless if a patient later complains. You need to write sufficient to ensure that you can efficiently assess the patient from the notes at the next appointment, that all key findings are noted and that, should a problem arise months or years later, the notes will support you and enable you to defend, explain and justify your actions and the care you provided.

Do you ever wonder why a patient who has not changed address has changed to your practice?

Is it your stunning good looks, your sartorial elegance, your winning smile, your sympathetic understanding of human nature, or your engaging conversation? Or could it be because you are a good GP?

Is it simply because you are local, easily accessible or have you been highly recommended by other patients? It is well worthwhile trying to establish what may have led to the patient joining the practice.

Ask a sensitive question or two. Perhaps there is dissatisfaction with a previous GP. What makes the new patient think that you can succeed where another GP has failed?

Think about asking:

- why the patient has changed GP
- what the patient has been told about the current physical state and any diagnoses that have already been made
- dates of treatment and treatments given.

What do you do when a patient comes to see you after treatment with another GP has been unsuccessful?

This can be very tricky. No one likes to be critical of a fellow professional. Perhaps the patient will ask you what you think about the treatment that has been provided previously. In these circumstances your primary obligation is to explain **current treatment needs** by assessing the current physical status.

The GP should recommend treatment. There is no requirement for a GP to make a judgement about any suggestion of negligence concerning a previous GP.

☢ This does not mean you have to be dishonest to a patient to protect a colleague. You have responsibility to the patient and to the GMC not to conceal poor or questionable care.

However, that does not mean jumping to conclusions about the circumstances under which particular diagnoses were reached or treatments undertaken.

Avoid getting drawn into a difficult situation. Don't guess why a GP undertook a particular course of treatment – you were not present at the time of the original history, examination and diagnosis. You cannot tell what signs were present at the time of the original consultation.

You should explain that you are not in a position to make a comment on why the previous GP treated the patient in a particular way.

Should you need to know about previous treatment for any reason, write to or telephone the GP. Do not make 'off the cuff' remarks about particular approaches to treatment. Casual or unguarded remarks may lead to the launch of a complaint against the previous practitioner. It could be your comments that set the whole thing off and you might then become entangled in any subsequent actions and be required to justify your remarks.

Your priority is to agree a successful course of treatment with the patient.

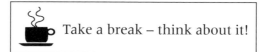 Take a break – think about it!

FINALLY

Do your records reflect well on you?

Make sure all the GPs in the practice can answer the following questions:

- Do the notes tell you everything you need to know about the patient's condition?
- If another GP treats this patient using these notes, would they be legible and comprehensible?
- If the notes were all you had, to defend a claim from several years earlier, would they be adequate?
- If your reputation depended on these notes, would you be OK?

PERSONAL RELATIONSHIPS WITH PATIENTS

The healthcare professions provide a unique window on the distress and suffering of patients and GPs develop a close physical and personal relationship with their clients.

Patients often return to see the GP many times and they see him or her not only as an expert in treating their symptoms, but also as someone in whom they can confide their anxieties and thoughts.

In consequence, patients often see their GP as their friend, and the relationship may be reciprocated. There is nothing unprofessional in such a relationship and there is no reason why a GP cannot continue to treat a patient who is regarded as a friend and indeed they may meet socially.

> ☑ The GMC document *Good Medical Practice* makes clear that the roles of patient and of friend should be kept clearly separated.

Such a relationship does, however, bring with it inherent potential dangers for the GP. It is sometimes difficult to ensure that the relationship is a purely social one and that it should have no influence on professional opinion.

Of course, a much greater problem emerges when a GP and a patient form an emotional or a sexual relationship.

Every practitioner knows and understands the problems that this causes and some GPs have suffered at the hands of

> ☢ The GMC guidance is quite clear and emphasises that it is a professional duty of the GP, absolutely, to avoid placing him or herself in such a position, and also to avoid any behaviour that might be construed as in any way inappropriate.

patients who have 'blown the whistle', usually when such a relationship comes to an end.

All professional bodies offer similar advice in such circumstances. They instruct that any practitioners who find themselves becoming emotionally or sexually involved with a patient **must** end the professional relationship immediately.

The patient must be treated by another GP. There should be no circumstances where it could appear that the patient was receiving clinical care at the same time as any personal interaction beyond the purely social.

Despite all that good advice, inevitably, emotional and physical relationships do develop between GP and patients. If it is discovered and reported to the GMC, there will be a hearing of the professional conduct committee (PCC).

It is likely that the penalty, handed down by the PCC, will be very harsh.

The circumstances in which these sorts of relationship develop are often complex. The emotional distress and damage to other personal and professional relationships is often so great that GPs finding themselves in these situations are more likely to need support and a sympathetic ear, rather than disapprobation.

It often falls to the Local Medical Committee, other senior colleagues or to the medical defence organisation adviser to provide that support and assistance.

Sometimes a GP will become aware of advances made by a patient. In such circumstances the GP should not make light of it or ignore it. Be sure to take definitive action in the event that the patient makes an inappropriate comment or action.

It is generally best to make a clear statement to the patient warning them that such a comment or action is unacceptable or, if serious, advising them that they should find another GP.

In these circumstances a proportion of patients will be apologetic or claim that the comment or action was misunderstood.

If the GP does decide to continue to treat the patient, it should be made entirely clear that if there is any repeat of the behaviour, the professional relationship with the patient will be terminated immediately.

A comprehensive note should be placed in the patient record describing the nature of the inappropriate behaviour, the warning given to the patient and the ultimatum about any further misbehaviour. In some circumstances the only action appropriate might be to remove the patient from the practice list altogether.

Sometimes dealing with the issue in writing is easier and in keeping a record on file!

A letter might say something like:

'In the surgery today you made comments (did something) that I found wholly unacceptable. Your advance was neither solicited nor acceptable.

'In order for us to have a professional working relationship and for me to continue providing your medical care I must emphasise that you must not behave in any way inappropriately.

'Our relationship must remain entirely professional. If you make any further advance I shall have no alternative but to terminate the care that I provide for you.'

It is important to remain firm and resolute, to ensure that all interactions are carefully recorded.

Notify any professional colleagues in the practice of what has happened, in case you need to seek their help, for example by transferring the patient to them.

WHISTLEBLOWING

Whistleblowing is a horrible term. It conjures up unpleasantness and, however deserved it may be, the idea of 'grassing' on a colleague, feels more at home in an episode of The Bill.

However, there are very good reasons why, sometimes, it is necessary to take action:

- A GP whose standard of practice is poor may well injure a patient. Supporting a colleague is fine but it should not be at the expense of the wellbeing of patients. The reputation of the whole profession may be damaged by a practitioner whose treatment is hazardous.

- Professional indemnity costs are based on the number and value of claims made against GPs. If substandard practitioners, making mistakes, are sued, the costs associated with their lack of competence will have to be spread across all practitioners, the vast majority of whom are of the highest calibre.

> ☢ The punishment for knowingly ignoring poor practice may be as harsh as that applied to the practitioner whose standards are in question.

- A GP knowing that a fellow practitioner is providing a poor standard of practice and putting patients at risk exposes themselves to risk. If it is discovered that a GP has practised whilst unfit or inadequately skilled to do so, and it comes to light that you knew, you will find yourself in front of the General Medical Council.

Of course, if you become aware that a colleague is performing badly he or she may be in desperate need of help. What should be done to help? It really all depends on your relationship with the practitioner in question.

You might consider the following:

- Talk to the practitioner yourself. If you do, there is a risk that you will be confronted with an aggressive response and a non-preparedness to discuss any problems at all. You could also find yourself in a difficult position if he or she seeks your help and places you in a position where you effectively have to monitor subsequent work. Tricky!

- Involve a senior colleague, usually through the LMC. Sometimes when confronted by a peer in age and seniority, the practitioner will acknowledge the problems.
- Contact your defence organisation and seek advice. Sometimes having someone independent with whom to discuss the matter is very helpful.
- Report the GP to the General Medical Council.

> The Health Committee of the General Medical Council has been very supportive in the past and their objective has always been, wherever possible, to help the GP to recover and to facilitate and expedite a return to practice. It remains to be seen whether the new unified arrangements are as good.

In some cases poor practice is the result of physical illness or emotional or psychiatric disorders. In such cases it is very important to ensure that the practitioner receives help quickly.

At the end of the day you may have to wrestle with your conscience. But the decision is not that hard. If you do nothing, it could lead to damage to patients, financial and professional damage to you and your colleagues, and you may end up in trouble yourself! It really isn't worth it.

CHAPERONES

During the course of many medical procedures patients may be required to remove clothing and submit themselves to intimate examinations.

Many treatments involve a physical closeness on the part of the GP or other healthcare professional. In such circumstances, where treatment is provided perfectly properly and to the highest standards, it may still be open to being misconstrued.

For that reason, healthcare professionals, for their own protection and for the reassurance of patients, are moving towards having chaperones available during any examination that is of a personal nature.

Some practitioners are opposed to the practice, fearing that privacy is lost, that there are difficulties in finding suitable chaperones and that there are not inconsiderable cost implications.

> Allegations involving same-sex inappropriate behaviour are very rare. Does that mean they don't happen?

However, the more general view is that chaperones are valuable in a number of situations:

- where the patient is of the opposite sex to the practitioner
- where clothing is removed and particularly where the more personal areas of the body may be partly or wholly exposed
- where treatment involves close physical contact
- where a patient asks for a chaperone
- where the GP feels that his or her own safety may be compromised without a chaperone.

Letting patients know chaperones are available may be done, in line with current recommendations, by having a notice in the waiting area stating that arrangements can be made for a chaperone to be in attendance on request. In addition, a similar notification can be placed in the practice booklet.

Sources of chaperones may either be members of staff (in circumstances where there are suitable staff that are available for such duties) or friends or relatives of the patient.

There has been discussion about:

- whether the chaperone should be able to see what is being done or whether it is adequate simply to hear any exchanges between patient and clinician
- whether a chaperone should be in the room in which the treatment is being provided or whether an open consulting room door and a receptionist sitting in a nearby (say) waiting area is adequate.

Opinions vary. We think that, in the current climate, it is adequate for a chaperone to be in the same room but separated from the patient and healthcare professional by (say) a curtain, so that it is possible to hear rather than see what is happening.

> ☑ The chaperone is present not to 'catch anyone out' but for reassurance.

> ☺ Would it be adequate for a chaperone (such as a receptionist) to be in an adjacent room provided that they are able to hear, clearly, what is being said?

This advice is on the basis that it seems extremely unlikely that, if a healthcare professional were to act in an unprofessional manner, the patient would not make some sort of comment that the chaperone would hear. However, depending on the patient, an in-sight view might be the answer.

If the patient requests that the chaperone observes what is being done, the practitioner would normally agree. In these cases the chaperone might be placed in a position where the view was general rather than specific, particularly when intimate areas are being examined.

Staff, in the role of chaperone, should fully understand the need for confidentiality of the same standard as that applied by the practitioner.

The whole practice team has a duty of confidentiality. However, the use of relatives or friends does pose a problem of confidentiality.

For example, if a patient attends a GP for treatment for (say) a skin condition, the agreement of the patient for the friend or relative to act as chaperone should only be assumed to be for the specific treatment for which consent has been given.

The GP, in this example, should not discuss medication or previous gynaecological history or issues surrounding other family members in the presence of the chaperone. Such a conversation should occur at the beginning or end of treatment, before there is any proximity between client and GP, and before the chaperone enters the room (or after he or she has left).

CONSENT

Under normal circumstances if a GP offers a patient a chaperone and it is refused, the GP should make a clear note of the refusal in the record. If a GP wishes a chaperone to be present for his or her own reassurance, then the patient must consent. If the patient refuses consent in circumstances where a GP has concerns, the practitioner should consider whether he or she should continue with the treatment un-chaperoned.

A chaperone may be of either sex. If the patient brings a friend or relative, clearly their choice will lead to a presumption of acceptability and they should then indicate whether there are any circumstances where their chaperone should not be admitted.

For the practitioner, it is acceptable to offer a chaperone of either sex (which could for example be another practitioner). The patient would, of course, have the right to reject a particular person as unacceptable.

Although chaperones provide reassurance and support for patients, they are also very important for the safety of the practitioner. A career can be placed in jeopardy by a groundless allegation of unprofessional treatment.

Although the idea of chaperones has not been popular with some practitioners, they can provide a crucial level of safety in some cases.

A practitioner should not be afraid to refuse to provide treatment if they feel vulnerable with a particular patient and there is no chaperone available.

✍ More and more healthcare is being delivered by clinical professionals, not just GPs. All of the healthcare professions will have to address this issue and it is likely that chaperones will soon be the rule rather than the exception.

DOMICILIARY VISITING

Even after the complications of the new GMS contract, some GPs still do home visiting!

It has its advantages. In genuine cases where patients are too ill to be seen in the surgery or are otherwise incapacitated, it allows them to be seen quickly and efficiently. However, there are some possible hazards and the GP should consider them before venturing into someone's house.

The greatest hazard is of course the risk of exposure to allegations of inappropriate behaviour occurring whilst in the patient's home. GPs have been exposed to this risk since the very first home visit took place and some have fallen foul of serious allegations.

Though it is difficult to avoid all risks it is possible to minimise them using a simple checklist of considerations before deciding to cross the threshold:

1 Do you know the patient seeking the visit? If it is a longstanding patient, you know him or her well and you are content that it is safe to go, there is probably no problem. You may not want to attend the home of a new patient on your own.
2 Have you done a visit before? If the request is part of an ongoing treatment, the visit will probably be safe.
3 Have you got any reason to be concerned about the visit? Concerns may exist because the patient has been 'flirty' in the past, or because you will find yourself alone with a patient in circumstances where, following any subsequent allegation, everyone says that it was obvious that you were taking a risk.
4 Are there any alarm bells ringing? Never ignore your own sixth sense. If you think it is a risk, don't do it on your own!

So, you decide to do a home visit and you find yourself alone in a house with a patient who is naked, lying in bed and has ideas that are not entirely medical. What do you do?

The answer is that you should have done and should do the following:

1 If you get a request for a home visit and you decide to go, make sure that the **request is documented** and that your staff member(s) **know that the request was made**.

2 If you are visiting a house where there is the remotest possibility that you could be compromised, tell the patient that you want him or her to have a relative, neighbour or friend present as a chaperone. It is usually reasonable to say that you cannot visit without such a prior arrangement. If you get to the house and there is no chaperone, you should leave, making a note of all the events.

3 If the patient is unwell but you feel that you could be compromised, you should not leave before you have made an assessment of the patient to ensure that they do not need immediate treatment.

4 Consider taking your own chaperone.

5 If you find yourself in a house, on your own, with a patient who shows any signs of misbehaviour, stop immediately, leave and make detailed notes of what happened and what you did when the patient behaved inappropriately.

☑ Don't forget that contemporaneous notes are still regarded as a good basis for a defence.

Always write extra notes in any situation where there may be concerns.

☢ Between a quarter and a sixth of all complaints about doctors relate in some way to visiting. It is clearly an important issue. Be careful, irrespective of whether you hate being called out or you find visiting an interesting part of the traditional medical practice approach to patients.

LOCUMS AND RISK

However committed you are to saving lives, the time will come when you want a day off to go to the cricket, the football, the school sports day, the rugby, visit relatives, go shopping or to some more exotic hobby like bungee jumping or morris dancing. See, you do have a life!

Alternatively, your other half may have presented you with an ultimatum: either go on holiday or deal with the divorce.

Basically, there is no discussion. It is time to get a locum. Easy, you may think; give the local locum agency a ring and fix it. Wrong!

It is not difficult to get a locum, but very difficult to get the right locum. Get the wrong person and they can screw up your practice, cause you to miss your quality targets, leave you having to deal with complaints and may bring the practice into disrepute if they are involved in an allegation of negligence.

> The locum will be acting in your stead.
>
> Whatever happens, if the locum does not perform well, it will rub off on you.
>
> One brush with a rude or abrupt locum may tarnish not only the GP's reputation but that of the whole practice.

There is very little data about locums. The Audit Commission did a report some years ago and it said the following:

- On a typical day in the NHS 3500 doctors will be working as locums in England and Wales – it is more now!
- The annual cost of locums is £200 million (surely much more than that now).
- About 10% of staffing costs in Trusts goes towards the costs of locums.
- About 70% of long-term locums between the ages of 35 and 55 have qualified overseas.
- The single greatest factor why overseas doctors become locums was because they couldn't find a permanent job, but that's changing. Now becoming a locum can be a career.

112

- Among UK-qualified locums, the greatest factor was to be able to combine work and the domestic agenda.

The Audit Commission concluded:

> Whilst there was no evidence that 'the care from a locum was of a lower standard than care from permanent staff', it did recommend 'a tightening up of the appointment and supervision of locums together with enforcing arrangements for performance review'.

This, of course, was before Shipman, Dame Janet Smith, the GMC tightening its rules and the development of revalidation and appraisal.

These days you need to be very careful when appointing a locum.

Here are the top 20 things you need to think about and get sorted:

1 Are planned absences from the practice agreed as part of surgery policy and will they be covered by other practice GPs or by locums?
2 How are locums appointed? Can you demonstrate that it is a monitored and audited process?
3 What steps do you take to be sure that their practise is safe and up-to-date?
4 Do they comply with PCT requirements?
5 Have you inspected the:
   - GMC practising certificate
   - defence organisation certificate.
6 Did you use a locum agency? Why that agency?
7 Do you know on what basis the agencies' locums are recommended?
8 Did the locum have testimonials and references?
9 Is the locum appointed by the GP who will be away or by the whole practice?
10 How will the locum's knowledge and experience be verified?
11 Will the locum's performance be reviewed by anyone? Who and how?
12 Do the patients have any involvement in the selection of a locum?
13 Do you have any information about the locum's admissions policy?
14 How will you be able to monitor the locum's prescribing activity?
15 Does the locum have a Professional Development Portfolio showing his postgraduate activities and, if so, have you seen it?
16 Is the locum's practice compared with practice indices?
17 Will the locum be expected to do visits? Do they understand the practice chaperone policy?

18 What is the reporting mechanism to monitor the locum's work?
19 Does the locum do work outside normal surgery activity (e.g. minor surgery) and if so are they approved?
20 Do you have a locum pack to familiarise the locum with the practice, policies, investigations forms, access to specialist services, etc?

MANAGING PATIENT EXPECTATIONS

In the words of Charles Dickens, patients have *Great Expectations*.

Over the last two decades we have moved into a seven-day-a-week, 24-hour-a-day, 'I need it now' culture, where patients have clear expectations of what they want and when they want it.

It can be the cause of considerable problems for practices when patients believe that GPs can offer treatments or achieve outcomes that are not possible.

Misleading articles in magazines or gossip may have led the patient to believe that a particular form of treatment is available, or likely to be successful, when it may be completely inappropriate or still a glimmer in a test tube in a laboratory in the USA.

GPs should not assume that patients understand anything about medicine. It is frequently the case that even simple procedures are not understood or are misunderstood by patients seeking treatment.

Increasing expectations are not confined to clinical issues. They include availability of parking, the comfort and privacy of the waiting area, the expectation of confidentiality when dealing with the receptionist and the

> ☢ Complaints and claims frequently arise because the GP fails to meet expectations.
>
> The description of diagnosis and treatment must be made absolutely explicit at the first consultation.

> ✎ If, at the outset, it is obvious that the patient has expectations you cannot meet, tell the patient, shake hands and let them go!

level of courtesy and friendliness afforded to them by the GP as well as by practice staff.

A number of common problems arise within the 'expectation zone', such as treatment of a nature or complexity that is beyond the GP:

- The request for treatment is in such a way or in a particular sequence that the GP does not feel is clinically acceptable or reasonable.
- Patient seeks appointment times that are unavailable, e.g. outside normal practice opening hours (an increasing challenge for the practice).
- Circumstances where the patient appears rude, aggressive or generally unpleasant or is simply someone that the GP really does not want to treat.

Furthermore, those practice policies that will impinge upon the patient's treatment should be made clear. These include:

- arrangements for making and cancelling appointments
- information about the necessary duration of appointments
- expectations, when appropriate, about what will be accomplished at each appointment.

Whatever it is, 'tell it early and tell it often'. Perception is everything. How you see it may not be how the patient sees it.

Look at it this way:

GP	Patient
Reasonable clinical standard	Does it match expectations?
Reasonable outcome	How long will it take?
Quality treatment	Will it hurt?
Notification of any standards that cannot be met	Will I be cured?

Matching what the GP can deliver against what the patient hopes for is the trick to ensure a minimum risk of disappointment, failure and possible litigation.

The condition of the practice is also a potent generator of expectation. The right premises can be reassuring for the patient:

- Are the premises well maintained?
- Are waiting area seats adequate?
- Are the magazines in good condition and recently published?
- Is there adequate facility for privacy and confidentiality?

- Are the toilet facilities adequate, clean and of a good quality?
- Are the consulting rooms efficient and comfortable looking?
- Are there facilities to notify patients of delay in appointments?
- Are brochures available for patients? Are they well presented and do they include information about:
  - the practice
  - telephone numbers
  - the GP(s) and staff
  - the types of services that are provided
  - any specialist services or services outside General Practice, e.g. acupuncture, osteopathy, nutrition
  - public transport and parking arrangements
  - the provision of care in an emergency
  - treatment exclusions
  - the policy (if any) if an appointment is missed or cancelled without adequate warning.

STAFF

Staff are the shop window of the practice. Consider carefully whether the front-line practice staff are the best advocates or driving patients away!

It is exceedingly difficult to smile continuously and be permanently pleasant, particularly if it is the end of a long day or there is trouble at home. Reception staff, in particular, need help and support to get through difficult days. They are the staff most likely to have trouble with difficult patients – more than nurses and GPs do. Consider their training needs. Find out whether the receptionist is the perfect receptionist. If they are they will:

- act courteously and with a friendly manner
- be able to act as a patient friend, adviser and supporter
- be able to act as an ambassador for the practice
- be able to negotiate and to have management skills
- be good on the telephone
- be dressed in a professional manner, clean and smart.

> ☺ Find out for yourself. Take 30 pence out of the petty cash, walk down the road to the call box and phone your practice up. See how helpful your receptionist is. You might just get a surprise.

If the answer is 'yes' to all of that – hang onto them. You have the perfect receptionist!

All obvious and basic? Yes, of course they are, but no receptionist will be rude or off-hand to the GP or practice manager. Sometimes they are not so nice and lovely to the patients.

CAN YOUR STAFF DEFUSE COMPLAINTS?

All the evidence is that if a complaint is handled quickly and professionally it is unlikely to escalate. Does your receptionist know what to do? Can they avoid disturbance and upset to other patients? Is any training necessary?

BAD DEBTS

Bad debts may be a problem for you if you treat private patients or provide services to businesses. If they are, do you have a policy for managing them? Issues will include:

- Is the sum outstanding actually worth claiming for the hassle involved?
- Is it substantial? If you are faced with a refusal to pay are you ready for a fight?
- If you can't get paid, is it because there is a perception that the treatment has been unsuccessful or of an inadequate standard? Are you certain that you should try to recover the sum?

> ✍ Remember
> Make it easy to pay and you'll probably get paid.

It is very important that each case is managed on its merits. Negotiation and personal conversation is easy to do and may help you get to the root of a problem if there is one. The small claims court is cheap and easy to use. Think about the use of a debt collecting agency.

PATIENT SURVEYS

Your services are excellent. They are universally popular and they meet all your patient needs.

> ☺ Patient questionnaires are cropping up throughout health-care and they are not all complete rubbish!

You know that, don't you? Oh really? Perhaps you should consider a patient questionnaire. Aside from the satisfaction of knowing you are right, a patient questionnaire is now worth quality points! Well worth doing.

Sometimes important changes occur because of patient observations that you may not have thought of.

If you decide to try one – and pretty well everyone is – make sure you include:

☑ In the new GMS contract there are 40 points up for grabs for a patient survey. Easy, get a helpful pharma-rep' to sort it out for you! There are two questionnaires that have been accredited: one called Improving Patient Questionnaire (IPQ) developed by Exeter University and the other the General Practice Assessment Questionnaire (GPAQ), developed by the National Primary Care Research and Development Centre in Manchester.

- a review of services provided
- the opportunity for patients to comment on services they might like to see
- the attitude of all staff, including the medical and clinical staff
- the ways the practice could be improved.

RISK AND FINANCE

FINANCIAL RISK MANAGEMENT

Standards of accounting in practices took a big leap forward following the NHS reforms in the early 1990s and the introduction of fundholding. As GPs became responsible for a higher percentage of the healthcare budget a higher standard of accounting and accountability was required.

In today's working environment, practice-based budgets are likely to become more common and once again the standards of accounting for public money are turned up another notch.

☢ The trouble with publishing web links is – they change! In general if you try a link and it doesn't work, try again using the link up to the first slash (/) and then navigate from the choices on the page.

Sorry, but that's technology for you!

If you are a real anorak and want to sound like you know a bit about finance at the next PCT meeting – here are some web links that will delight and entertain you:

- Department of Health (2002) (updated) *Corporate Governance Framework for Primary Care Trusts*:
  www.doh.gov.uk/pct/2002/corpgovframeworkmanualaug02.pdf.
- Department of Health (1996) *Directions on Financial Management* HSG (96) 12:
  www.info.doh.gov.uk/doh/Coin4.nsf/
  12d101b4f7b73d020025693c005488a9/
  7897ddded1c3b2d1002564b90049fb69/$FILE/12HSG.PDF.

- Department of Health (2002) *Internal Audit Standards for the National Health Service*:
  www.info.doh.gov.uk/doh/rm5.nsf/
  e38b211034b364b500256735003e21ae/
  5e40cf2557aa4c8e002569ee00405182/$FILE/ATTW83XJ/
  GIAS%20Standard%20final%2015%206%2002.pdf.
- Department of Health (1994) *Codes of Conduct and Accountability* EL (94) 40:
  www.info.doh.gov.uk/doh/rm5.nsf/
  b7546ce4a0608579002565c4003bf709/
  c76450804533b73300256a1800532077/$FILE/
  code%20of%20conduct-accountability.doc.
- Department of Health (1999) *Governance in the New NHS: Controls Assurance Statements 1999/2000: Risk Management and Organisational Controls* HSC 1999/123:
  www.info.doh.gov.uk/doh/coin4.nsf/
  12d101b4f7b73d020025693c005488a9/
  8cb87ab15a090349002567780031bbe3/$FILE/123HSC.PDF.
- Department of Health (2003) *Delivering Excellence in Financial Governance*:
  www.doh.gov.uk/financialgovernance/deliveringexcellence.pdf.
- Department of Health (2003) *Delivering Excellence in Financial Governance: The statutory role of the Director of Finance*:
  www.doh.gov.uk/financialgovernance/2statutory.htm.
- Department of Health (2002) *Code of Conduct for NHS Managers*:
  www.doh.gov.uk/nhsmanagerscode/codeofconduct.pdf.
- Department of Health (2002) *Example: Reservation of Powers to the Board and Delegation of Powers*:
  www.ntwha.nhs.uk/Board_Papers/a3402/
  Reservation%20%20Delegation%20of%20Powers.pdf.
- Department of Health (annual publication) *Manuals for Accounts*:
  http://tap.ukwebhost.eds.com/doh/finman.nsf/
  FAQs?OpenView&Start=1&Count=1000&ExpandView.
- Department of Health (1998) *Countering Fraud in the NHS* HSC 1999/208:
  www.info.doh.gov.uk/doh/coin4.nsf/
  12d101b4f7b73d020025693c005488a9/
  be905af54928591c002567ef003b8ce2/$FILE/208.PDF.

 OK, so in the hope you've got that out of your system – let's look at the practice.

FINANCIAL RISK MANAGEMENT FOR THE PRACTICE IS NO MORE THAN COMMON SENSE

Here are the basics:

1 Is all income routinely monitored?
2 Do the practice partners understand the accounting system?
3 Does the practice produce regular monthly management accounts and are they formally noted and adopted by all the partners?
4 Is all the expenditure in the practice routinely monitored and always authorised before the event?
5 If budgets, even nominal budgets, are cascaded, how can you protect against careless overspending?
6 When items are procured, is a value for money (VFM) exercise always followed?

VFM?

Value for money (VFM) can be evaluated in several ways: VFM over the long term; VFM evaluated against current ways of doing things; VFM in the sense of stopping doing something one way and starting doing it in another. VFM is not about cheapest, or fastest. The key is the evaluation of the word 'value' in the context of the plan.

Value may mean paying more in the short term, in order to gain value in the longer term.

For those anoraks really interested in VFM, there is a great book, written by John Marriotti, *Shape Shifters*, published by VNR (ISBN 0-442-02559-9).

VFM is described as a pentangle, made up of quality, service, cost, speed and innovation.

The pentangle is drawn like this:

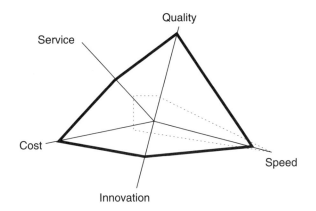

As you can see, there is a thick black line that joins the key components. The closer the line is to the name of the component, the more important it is.

This model describes a service that needs to be:

- fast
- not specially innovative
- cheap to acquire
- with a high level of quality
- without much service required to back it up.

You will see the dotted line describes something quite different! A fast cheap, basic, service. This is a simple way to get your head the right way round when evaluating what VFM means in your context.

Draw a pentangle to evaluate VFM on four projects:
- a new examination couch for the surgery
- resurfacing the car park
- a car leasing system for district nurses
- electronic sphygmomanometers for five surgeries plus the nurses room.

See how the shapes change?

Use the evaluation pentangle for your plans. Remember, the idea is not to create diagrams, it is to create VFM.

TIME FOR SOME FINANCE STUFF

☑ ☢ ☺ ✍ Who does all this finance stuff? Normally it is in the purview of the Practice Manager. Their financial literacy is vital. No matter how good they are at everything else, they have to be good at the 'numbers thing'.

Also, at least one practice partner should take responsibility for over-seeing the finance function. This is not a job for a keen amateur. Make sure whoever does the job – does the job! Properly!

Finally, the practice needs to appoint a good firm of accountants, with experience of the NHS and primary care.

All practices should routinely produce the following.

A balance sheet

This is an overall position statement setting out the value of the practice, its assets, its income and expenditure.

A 'profit and loss account'

Profit and loss is an expression commonly used in the business community and hardly needs a definition.

In the wider NHS, where profits are not made, it is probably easier to think of it as income and expenditure.

Profits might be seen as managing surpluses or losses on activity, man-power and finances. However, the practice can, and should, make a profit, or surplus at year end.

A cash flow forecast

Cash flow is seen as the life blood of most businesses and a practice is no different. Companies that trade at the margins of profitability can sometimes keep going for longer than they should because they have a positive, regular and healthy cash flow. It is also true that very profitable organisations have crashed because their cash flow has been poor and they have run out of money.

The practice will have income in the normal sense, 'draw-down' arrange-ments with the PCT and reimbursement arrangements with the PCT.

Think box

Primary care is increasingly encouraged to work creatively with partners outside the NHS, organisations such as social services and some others in the private and voluntary sector. If an initiative is joint funded, or to come from the newly 'pooled budget' arrangements with social services, think about timescales.

The public sector financial year runs from April to March. Is that the same for everyone you are involved with? Are different accounting arrangements within different organisations likely to be a problem?

A combination of these sources of income can complicate cash flow reports. The flow of cash through the practice should be monitored very closely as it will have to be balanced off against the payment commitments; when the practice is likely to be called upon to make payments and when they are to expect receipts.

All this gets turned on its head if there is an unexpected demand on services, such as in the winter months, and there is not enough cash in the system to pay the bills.

Keeping up to date with what is happening

Make sure reporting arrangements allow for regular updates of financial situation.

Don't be shy about circulating budgets. People have got to know where they are – good or bad. Transparency helps to avoid insolvency.

Regular reports are called **management accounts**.

They should be produced regularly and consistently, in the same format so that it is easy to identify trends; they must be detailed enough to be interesting and helpful, but not so detailed as to be confusing.

Computer technology can be used to employ accounting packages that are

Software is cheap and misunderstandings expensive. Graphs, bar charts and graphics can compare last month with this month and the year to date with target – easy! Simpler than a page of numbers.

capable of displaying complex information in graphical and simple-to-understand ways.

☺ **Exercise**

How financially literate are the people you work with? It's OK not to be an accountant! Honest! The important thing is that reports are regular and everyone who has responsibility understands what's going on. Practice principals, clinicians and managers may not be entirely populated with people who feel comfortable with the numbers.

However, the evidence is clear. Organisations that share financial information with all staff (budgetholders or not) do better with financial management than the ones who don't.

Develop a system for financial reporting that is accurate, not threatening to non-finance people and can be produced easily. What does technology have to offer?

INCOME AND EXPENDITURE FORECAST

A PCT is forbidden, by statute, to make a 'loss' – or in the language of the public sector, spend more than its allocation. However, a practice might easily slip into a loss-making period.

Start-up projects, using pump-priming funds, the sort that will require a business case, may legitimately not have their income matching their expenditure.

☢ In a new project, be sure to be realistic with projections and if there is an excess of expenditure over income – don't hide it.

The key is to be realistic.

The shortfall may be picked up elsewhere. Be careful to make realistic projections and if there is an excess of expenditure over income – don't hide it. The key is to be realistic.

Decide over what period you can realistically forecast in detail. In the world of business, high volume, high turnover activity is measured in weeks and months. Low volume, low turnover in months and years.

Think of a forecast as a photograph of how you see activity taking place; a careful picture of the detail up-close and a snap of what the view might be, from further away.

The income flow forecast

In business this would be called the cash flow forecast – it's all the same. The forecast is simply a chronological list of expected expenditure deducted from anticipated income.

The calculation is done month by month, through the year. Include all expenditure and remember leases are not free – include them.

Here is an example of a cash flow chart with some sample headings:

Sample cash flow chart (first year)

Month	1	2	3	4	5	6	7	8	9	10	11	12
Total income												
Opening balance (A)												
Initial investment/grants, etc.												
Income												
Asset disposal												
Interest on deposits												
Total income (B)												
Payments												
Purchase of lease/property												
Furniture/fittings												
Vehicles												
Materials												
Employees wages, tax/NI												
Training costs/conferences												
Rent/rates												
Fuel												
Telephone												
Post												
Printing/stationery												
Subscriptions/periodicals												
Public meeting costs/ promotion												
Repairs/maintenance												
Vehicle costs												
Travel												
Insurance												
Professional fees												
Loan/grant repayments												
Bank charges												
VAT												
Other expenses												
Total outgoings (c)												
Receipts, less payments for the month (D)												
(B) – (C) = (D)												

Cash remaining in the system
Sample cash flow forecast chart (years 2 & 3)

Year/Quarter	2/1	2/2	2/3	2/4	3/1	3/2	3/3	3/4
Receipts								
Opening balance (A)								
Initial investment/grants, etc.								
Income								
Asset disposal								
Interest on deposits								
Total receipts (B)								
Payments								
Purchase of lease/property								
Furniture/fittings								
Vehicles								
Materials								
Employees wages, tax/NI								
Training costs/conferences								
Rent/rates								
Fuel								
Telephone								
Post								
Printing/stationery								
Subscriptions/periodicals								
Public meeting costs/ promotion								
Repairs/maintenance								
Vehicle costs								
Travel								
Insurance								
Professional fees								
Loan/grant repayments								
Bank charges								
VAT								
Other expenses								
Total payments (c)								
Receipts, less payments for the month (D) (B) − (C) = (D)								
Cash remaining in the project								

Procurement

If the practice envisages the acquisition of any capital equipment, detail what it is and how its purchase is to be financed. Such items might include: computers, mobile phones, fax machines and office furniture. A plan might concern the development of buildings or extensions to existing premises.

EXERCISE

List all the capital items (costing more than £300) required in the first three years, including (in each case) how they will be purchased – lease, loan, cash, rent, etc.

Capital item	Initial cost	Time of anticipated purchase	Method of payment	Completion of loan, etc.

Plus:

• What is the procurement process for new items? Are items to be researched and selected, or is a specification to be drawn up and bids invited? Who is going to do it and by when?
• Where is the line of accountability?
• Draw up a complete list of the equipment the practice might procure in the year. Consider how they will be financed.

PHARMACY, FORMULARY AND CONSUMABLES

How are the pharmacy and arrangements for replenishing consumables to be handled and how are formulary decisions to be arrived at?

• Group purchase?
• Who's in charge?
• Accountability?
• Decisions and methodology of adding new drugs to the formulary.

> ☑ **Tip:**
> Three words to remember about stock control: quantity, value, frequency.

• Impact of NSF, NICE Guidelines and generic prescribing targets – how is progress against target reviewed?

In business this would be 'stock control' and the same approach is good for practices and other public sector projects. Stock control is good discipline.

Too much stock (or consumables) and valuable money is tied up unnecessarily. Too little and you run the risk of running out of something vital.

Consider reorder levels and lead-time for replenishment and minimum levels it is safe to operate at. High tech devices often come with expensive consumables to make them work. Be sure to make realistic estimates about the frequency and costs involved.

MANAGEMENT INFORMATION SYSTEMS

Things can go wrong in every organisation, it is no great sin. The sin is not knowing that something has gone wrong!

A simple way to describe management information systems is 'keeping a finger on the pulse'. An organisation is very much like a living thing. Progress is measured by the day and progress from one day to the next can be very different. Sometimes the business (and a practice is a business) will be fit and healthy and at other times it could be a bit under the weather. Diagnosing a sick organisation is the job of practice managers – the organisation's doctor! To make a diagnosis you need a list of symptoms – they are called management reports.

Reports will include:

• cash flow
• income
• expenditure
• activity levels.

Example management accounts

Sample headings

	Month 1	Month 2	Month 3
Employment costs			
Wages, salaries, etc.			
Training			
Premises			
Rent			
Rates/water			
Running costs			
Fuel			
Telephone			
Postage			
Printing			
Subscriptions			
Vehicles			
One-off start-up costs			
Repairs			
Insurance			
Professional fees			
Interest payments			
Bank charges			
Depreciation – vehicles			
Depreciation – other assets			
Other expenses			

FINANCIAL MANAGEMENT CRITERIA

Get this right and your practice won't wander too far off the straight and narrow! All of these headings are the responsibility of someone! The question is: who?

> ☺ It is becoming increasingly likely that the practice manager will be a partner.

Well, it could be an autocratic GP! More likely it is the partners group, or some group mandated by them. It might be the practice manager – reporting to the partners. There are a variety of approaches and from practice to practice this may vary. The important thing is to identify who is in charge – who to sack if it all goes wrong and who to give a big bonus to when it all goes right!

In the interests of governance – of which more later – there should be a clear line of responsibility and a reporting mechanism to ensure the job is being done. Finance control should never be left to a single individual.

	Yup	Doin' it	Err . . .

1 Define the hierarchy and process for ultimate financial responsibility in the organisation – individual, or group (for convenience, called here 'the partners').

2 Financial objectives for the organisation are clearly defined, approved by the partners.

3 Partner-level responsibility for financial management is clearly defined and is supported by clear lines of financial accountability throughout the organisation.

4 There are adequate audit arrangements overseeing all the financial aspects of the practice.

5 Standing financial instructions, based on the Department of Health model and updated to reflect current requirements, have been formally adopted by the practice and understood throughout the practice.

6 Financial risk management processes exist throughout the practice.

7 There is an effective and documented system of internal control for all financial management systems.

8 There is an adequately resourced, trained and competent finance function/person.

9 All employees, including clinicians, who are budgetholders are provided with adequate information, instruction and training on financial management.

10 The partners review the effectiveness of its system of internal control for financial management at least annually.

11 The partners receive regular reports on financial performance and activity. They are made aware of significant risks and determine and take appropriate action.

12 Internal audit provides an annual assurance to the partners on the effectiveness of practice's financial arrangements based on this standard.

13 The practice can demonstrate that it has done its reasonable best to meet its key financial objectives.

14 Arrangements are in place to appoint external auditors for annual audit and their report presented to the partners.

GETTING TO GRIPS WITH COMMUNICATION

We wonder how many readers remember what three-and-fourpence was? Three shillings and four pence, written 3/4d. Actually, it is nearly 17 pence in decimal coinage. Somehow, three-and-fourpence had a charm and individuality that we have lost. But we digress.

Apparently during a First World War campaign a beleaguered group of luckless soldiers were dug in, with the enemy all around. The commander saw that his only way to survive was to advance but he needed more troops to do it. So he sent a messenger to return as quickly as he could to the headquarters with the message, 'Send reinforcements, I'm going to advance.' The message relay arrangements resulted in the message being passed by word of mouth from messenger to messenger. When the message finally arrived at the Brigade Headquarters the final messenger was able to pass on the information to the Commanding Officer, 'Send three-and-fourpence, I'm going to a dance.'

Silly? Yes! But, it illustrates how easily communications can let us down and how easy it is for comments to be misunderstood.

Get the communication right and the chances are you will get the diagnosis right. The patient will go home reassured, understanding what they will have to do, knowing what to expect.

Communication is two-way. There is the information that the patient passes to the GP and the information that the GP passes to the patient – with quite a lot of chat in the middle.

> ☢ It is important to understand that breakdowns in communication are at the heart of most claims for negligence against healthcare professionals.

> Have a cup of coffee and think about the communications in your own practice – between the GPs, practice staff, the patients and each with each other. What do you get? Tower of Babel?

Accuracy is often the casualty. There is a world of difference between, for example, an acute pain and a chronic pain. Yet patients commonly mix the two words and the outcome could be an entirely wrong understanding on the part of the practitioner.

Here are some ideas to help improve communication during a consultation with a practitioner. Better communication equals lower risk. It has got to be good:

- Let the patient make the initial running. Allow them to voice their concerns and explain their problems.
- Listen with genuine interest. Don't hold a pen, write notes or type onto the computer screen whilst they are talking to you. Concentrating on what is being told to you works wonders.
- Shut up. A study showed that doctors are completely unable (most of the time) to keep quiet for more than 13 seconds. If a silence develops whilst the patient is talking, keep quiet. The patient may often fill the gap with something more or useful or with greater clarity.
- Look for clues as the patient speaks to you:
  - Do they make eye contact?
  - Do they look anxious, sad or angry?
  - What is their breathing telling you?
  - Look at the facial expression and gestures.
  - Does their clothing tell you anything?
- Don't rush to judgement. Be prepared to challenge your initial conclusions.
- Ask yourself key questions:
  - What is the key problem that the patient is telling me about?
  - Why this patient?
  - Why at this time?
  Repeat back what they have said to you. This lets the patient correct anything that you may have got wrong or they haven't explained very well.
- Avoid techno-speak and jargon. Simple words may be misunderstood by even very bright people.
- Remember that you have a special place in the community. In the minds of many people you are a powerful figure. Don't sit behind a desk and surround yourself with medical equipment, books, papers, etc.

- Make it easy for the patient. Think about their lifestyle, intelligence and resources.
- Remember perception is everything.
- Look for 'non-verbal leakage' (what a terrible expression). The phrase means the need to spot the difference between what the patient says and what their non-verbal behaviour is telling you. Everyone has had a patient that says 'No I'm not depressed' whilst sitting, shoulders slumped, with a sad fixed expression and exuding gloom.
- Consider what your words will mean to the patient. 'Won't' means 'might', 'can't' means 'could' and 'shouldn't' means 'probably will'.
- It is sometimes helpful to speak in the plural to emphasise the 'we're all in this together' approach. Useful words are 'we', 'us' and 'together'.
- Have good leaflets to market, promote, explain and support what you have said. After outlining a series of exercises, a leaflet that emphasises what you have said is a great back-up. They should be neat, coloured if the exchequer will run to it and written in friendly English – not tatty little photocopies.

Leaflets can make a big difference to a practice. If you give every new patient a leaflet about the practice – who the staff are, their qualifications, the practice facilities, opening hours, etc. – the likelihood is that it will be retained and referred to.

> Consider the need to translate practice leaflets into other languages, for the benefit of patients whose first language is not English.

Leaflets about particular medical conditions are so useful and, again, provide excellent advertising. They need not cost a fortune: with desktop publishing so good these days, what you really need is a 10-year-old to do it for you – they are all computer wizards. Many pharma-companies supply them for free.

If you work with colleagues or practitioners from other disciplines, have you looked at the communication with them?

- How do you pass information? Not post-it notes stuck on windows and computer screens. There have been disasters when they have become detached and lost and messages have not reached the intended recipient.
- Do you actually have a process for ensuring relevant information, guidance and so on is passed around?
- Do you know what should be passed and what you will say when it is?
- What is likely to go wrong?

- Will a good communication system cost money?
- How will you know if it has worked?

Let's face it. Some GPs are really good at communicating with patients and others are, well, less good. Some are attentive, considerate and supportive whilst others are arrogant, self-opinionated and directive.

The latter group includes the 'GP knows best' group and they are much more likely to have a clinical negligence catastrophe. They will also damage their own reputations with their clients.

Leading practices are now creating **patient participation groups**. They are great:

- They will give you feedback on the services you provide.
- They will help you if you have difficulties with other clients or the local authorities.
- They will fund-raise for you if you want particular bits of equipment.
- They can publicise you in a way you can't and can help to build your practice.
- They will be your best allies if the going gets tough.

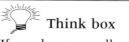 **Think box**

If you have a really good consultation with a patient who is absolutely thrilled with your care, it is probable that they will tell **one** other person, probably a relative.

If the consultation is awful they will tell **10** other people. Reputations spread, but the speed is up to you!

So communication is very important, between you and the patients, between you and the community, between you and your colleagues. It is worth the effort.

INFORMATION TECHNOLOGY AND RISK MANAGEMENT

Judging by the records that we see during the course of medical defence work, it would be jolly nice if GPs still did everything on paper records.

We know that computerised records are legible (if you allow for the appalling spelling) but

> Handwritten records have their advantages. They are not constrained by the limitations of any system. They tend to be written during a consultation whilst computerised records tend to be written after a consultation.

the pigeon-English, computer-speak abbreviations can be entirely confusing. And you don't ever see ridiculous entries like 'Miscellaneous disease – other', which one medical computer system generates if there is no option on offer to fit what the patient is actually suffering from.

However, handwritten notes are not good for audit or research. To be able to press a button and identify how many left-handed, aboriginal men have occupational backache at your practice can be useful and time-saving if your friendly local PCT requires it (though be careful of the confidentiality issues!).

GPs are required to use a coding system to record the diseases and disorders that they identify. The coding system does at least give a clue to incidence but some of the codes are truly bizarre. We are prepared to bet that not many doctors use the code for 'Struck by a falling Astronaut'.

Microsoft's Windows-based systems provide a good basis for most simple record keeping and are ideal for the single or small practice, although more comprehensive bespoke systems are available.

For the GP who is to IT what Pavarotti is to bricklaying, and who is not sure what to buy, it is essential to avoid seeking advice from the gifted amateur. You need a professional.

If you want a bespoke system you must develop a list of criteria that you require to be filled and a clear description of the system to be provided or designed, what it will do, what it will not do and whether and how it would link with other systems, such as those currently in use or development within the NHS.

As a general piece of advice you should be very careful about rushing into getting a system if the urge takes you. Hospitals and practices have a history of disasters, where large sums of money were wasted and huge amounts of time frittered away, trying to make an unworkable system work.

The best advice is always to use a system that someone else already has working and that you can see demonstrated to your own satisfaction before proceeding to buy one yourself.

The NHS National Programme for IT, the so-called NPfIT, is a £6.2 billion roll-out to connect 30 000 GPs, 500 Trusts and places of treatment and the medical records of 60 million UK citizens. And it is coming down your way, some day soon!

In time it will involve patient preference appointments, electronic prescribing, e-health patient records and histories and probably a healthcare entitlement card reader. It is the most ambitious IT project ever attempted, anywhere in the world.

Be sure what you invest in is NPfIT-compatible. If it's not, don't buy it and shoot the person trying to sell it to you.

That said, here are some more **Dos and Don'ts**:

- At the risk of repeating ourselves, do make sure that it meets any standards that are required by any relevant authorities and that it is compatible with any other systems with which it may be required to communicate, now **or in the future**. It must be compatible with the PCT system.
- Do make sure you know what you want. The all-singing, all-dancing Pentium 123XYZ may be brilliant but do you really **need** the specification or will something less spectacular (and cheaper) meet your requirements.
- **Futureproof** your machine. Make sure it does not have obsolescence built into it. It should be upgradeable, flexible and be capable of having the memory expanded. No one ever has enough memory.

- Don't forget your obligations under the Data Protection Act. If you have any questions, telephone the Registrar's office on 01625 545745.
- Think about confidentiality when you have records on the computer. Don't leave screens of information unattended. Don't forget to set up a password.
- Back up your files. If you lose data it may be irretrievable and it may cause havoc in your practice. The best advice is:
  - Back up data **every day**.
  - Rotate the back-up tapes or discs **every day for a week**.
  - Back up critical information **twice a day**.
  - You'll be pleased you took the advice **one day**!
- Don't make it easy for someone to steal your equipment. The local Crime Prevention Officer will be pleased to help.
- Don't get a virus. When you connect up your machine to the big electronic world, the first thing to do is install a reliable virus checker – Norton or McAfee or some such.

☢ Don't use an obvious password like your daughter's first name and don't give your password to anyone else (like the receptionist for instance).

However much you trust your receptionist, ask yourself how private detectives find out medical information about patients – it is available if the price is right!

☢ Don't allow staff to load games or any other software onto the practice PCs.

They take up memory space, they should not be used. They may introduce nasty viruses into your machine and anyway, how come they have time to play games?

- Fit a surge protector to the electrical supply for all your PCs. What is it? It is a device for flattening out spikes that occur in the electricity system so that a surge of electricity does not damage the delicate equipment in the PC. A surge can mean blank screens and misery. Or even worse, a blue screen and certain disaster. The device only costs a few pounds and is well worth the expense. Some also give you a few moments of reserve power – to back up your system in the event of a power cut.

Email is now ubiquitous. Increasingly it is being used for professional purposes, including referrals, educational exchanges and patient communications.

However, with these great benefits come some problems and the practice should be on top of them. Email systems are simple to use and therein lays one of their major weaknesses. It is easy to pass messages to a large number of people very quickly and those messages can include pictures and graphics.

A sign of things to come was heralded by a court case in the United States in 1999 when a merchant bank agreed a large out-of-court settlement with two of its employees because some staff had used the email system to circulate a bad-taste joke about African Americans.

The aggrieved staff reached for their lawyers and the company reached for its chequebook. The court decided that the employers are responsible for internal email traffic regardless of its origin. Since then, legal actions across the world have arisen from allegations about everything from sexual discrimination to breach of confidence, in organisations without proper email policies and planning.

> ☢ Some people try the trick of sticking a blank email into the file every so often so that they can add information at a later stage.
>
> It may fool people at a superficial level but if suspicion is raised, don't forget the experts and the 14-year-olds, who can work out just what you have done and when you did it.

If your practice were to become involved in a court case or an industrial tribunal, email is ready to provide another shock.

A legal device known as **discovery** can be used to force defendants to reveal every file, note and piece of paper they have that might be pertinent to the case.

Nothing can be hidden. Courts can look in your filing cabinets, your archives and on your hard disk too.

If they discover that you have deliberately erased emails or other electronic documents you may find yourself in contempt of court. Computer experts can find hidden 'history' and cache files in Windows$^©$ and other systems that can leave a trail of clues to what has been done to the files. Emptying the Recycle Bin does not mean gone for good.

If you are using email, and particularly if your system may have several users, you should consider setting up practice protocols and guidance fast.

Here are the rules:

1 Warn all staff with an on-screen message about the practice's rules for email.

2 Make it clear that email is **not** confidential and will be routinely monitored. Hammer home the fact that email is not a substitute for the kind of conversation that used to take place in the canteen, lavatory or lift.

3 Stamp out any digital gossip. Bar the transmission of personal mail, jokes, smutty material and non-business messages. Experience shows that you may be vulnerable for what any member of your staff does electronically.

4 Set up in-house e-instruction to make sure that staff understand the rules. Incorporate the policies into contracts of employment.

5 Install a programme that monitors email for key words and phrases to flag up offensive material.

6 Decide on archive policies. What will you keep, where, how long will you keep it and who will be responsible for it?

 VERY BIG HAZARD WARNING

Never, never, never, never, never, never, never, never, never, never, never, never, never open an attachment to an email that has the suffix .EXE unless it came from your mum or the priest.

And even then be suspicious.

These types of file are a commonly used vehicle for lunatics spreading viruses.

In fact it is wise not to open any email message if you have no idea who the sender is. These days it is possible to screw up your computer system with word processing files, jpeg picture files and all sorts of other material. A virus checker is the answer – the sort that updates itself to keep you free of the latest attacks from the bobble-hat brigade.

REVIEWING THE PRACTICE

How does your place look? The next section is about health and safety, but let's get started with spotting general hazards.

The only way to do a proper review is to do a risk management audit. It may sound difficult but it is really just common sense. The plan is to find out what can go wrong and to do something about it – before it does!

SEVEN STEPS FOR IMPLEMENTING A RISK MANAGEMENT SYSTEM

1 **Identify the key risk areas:** The trick here is to involve everyone in the practice. Speak to your staff and ask them where they think the risks are. Have a look at anything that may have gone wrong in the past, check previous insurer contacts if you have had any claims, review any patient complaints and, if possible, talk to patients.

> 😊 **Try this**
> If you have 15 minutes, try the Post-It Note Test.
> Give everyone some Post-Its and ask them to make a note and stick it on every dodgy plug, dangly wire, faulty window, etc. It might be a revelation to you.

2 **Identify key trigger events:** Look for trends. History can be a great guide. If it's happened before it may well happen again. Keep an eye out for national incidents – could they happen to you?

3 **Implement an incident reporting system:** Things go wrong everywhere. It is no sin unless you don't do anything about it. Make sure if any staff see a problem they feel comfortable to tell you about it. You need a no-blame culture. Near misses are particularly important. Furthermore, it is good to

learn from our mistakes but a whole lot better to learn from other people's.

4 **Investigate high-risk events:** When something does go wrong, investigate it immediately. Take action even if all the facts are not immediately to hand. Look for the cause and how to avoid a recurrence. If staff are involved, find out their view on what happened but remember that they may be cautious or feel threatened.

5 **Monitor and analyse reports for trends:** You may need an anorak for this. Spot incidents and near-misses that happen more than once. Risk management is about predicting what might go wrong. Be honest and, if necessary, self-critical.

6 **Implement changes in the practice as necessary:** No point in bothering with trends and all that if you are not going to make use of it. Make sure the practice staff understand why change is necessary.

7 **Education and feedback:** Most accidents occur out of ignorance. Make sure everyone knows what has been a problem and why it is no longer a problem.

You may be able to get further help from:

• the professional indemnity (defence) organisation
• the General Medical Council
• the local Primary Care Trust (but we wouldn't bet on it!)

. . . and this fabulous book!

Finally, if your review throws up a number of problems, use the risk formula to assess risk

$$\text{Risk} = (\text{Likelihood of hazard}) \times (\text{Severity of consequences})$$

$$\text{Risk factor*} = \text{Numerical representation of risk.}$$

*Where 1 is low and 5 is high, allocate a number between one and five to express the likelihood of the hazard and a number between 1 and 5 to measure the potential severity of the consequences. Multiply them together and use that as a numerical expression of relative risk.

What you need is a checklist for your buildings to make sure that there is nothing obvious that may cause you a problem. A building costs a lot of money to build and maintain and it is worth looking after even if only for the sake of making sure it contributes to your pension fund! More importantly, the public and the staff are in and out of the place, so it must be safe and meet the health and safety standards (more of this in the next chapter).

It is worth walking around the surgery and thinking about it from the perspective of the patients, adults and children, as well as the staff. Here is a list of the sort of things they should be looking for:

	OK	Not OK	Who will sort it	By when
The reception/waiting area				
• Is the entrance door easy for a patient to open?				
• Is there a disabled access?				
• Is the reception on one level?				
• If doors are fully glazed are there markings to indicate the presence of glass for partially-sighted patients?				
• Is glass in doors toughened or laminated?				
• Is part of the reception desk at a suitable height for patients in wheelchairs?				
• Is there a hearing loop for deaf patients?				
• Is there an area where a patient can speak in confidence to a receptionist?				
• Is the telephone situated such that patients waiting in reception cannot hear conversations with patients?				
• Are there sufficient chairs?				

	OK	Not OK	Who will sort it	By when
• Are patients kept informed of delays in being seen?				
• Are all parts of the waiting room visible to staff?				
• Is there adequate heating and ventilation?				

Consulting room
- Is the room of adequate size, ventilated and heated?

- Is the plinth appropriately located and suitably screened?

- If you use sharps, is the sharps box inaccessible to small children?

- Is the room equipped with a panic alarm?

- Is the floor safe?

- Is the lighting adequate?

- Is the décor of suitable colours for partially sighted patients?

- Are carpets free of frays and suitably fitted to avoid the risk of slipping or tripping?

- Are floors safe and not slippery?

	OK	Not OK	Who will sort it	By when

Toilets
- Do they meet requirements for disabled access?

- Is there an alarm for a patient unwell or immobile in the toilet?

- Can the toilet door be opened by a staff member from outside?

There you are. That should keep you going for a little while, but at least the surgery will have no obvious hazards that might end up costing you much more time and heartache.

HEALTH AND SAFETY 1

Increasingly, practitioners are working in groups and the surgeries from which they practice are becoming their biggest assets. The practice should be aware of health and safety

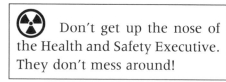 Don't get up the nose of the Health and Safety Executive. They don't mess around!

requirements, as they are complex and can relate to issues ranging from employment to cross-infection.

It is just possible that you might not be fully up to date with the health and safety regulations?

Well, here are the basics:

You should be aware of Section 2 of the Health and Safety at Work Act 1974, which details responsibilities for all people who work in the premises, whether employed, self-employed or the employer.

Failure to comply can lead to prosecution by the Health and Safety Executive (HSE). The responsible employer (that's you!) must provide and maintain a safe working environment with safe equipment and procedures in place.

It is not all one-way. Employees have responsibilities, too. They must have due regard to health and safety procedures and report anything that could compromise this to the person in charge (that means you as well!).

Health and safety legislation is becoming more risk-led. There is a specific duty placed on employers to assess the risks to which their employees are exposed.

'The requirement to assess risks may be general, as in the Management of Health and Safety at Work Regulations 1999, or specific, as in the Control of Substances Hazardous to Health Regulations (COSHH).

Under health and safety law the employer is required to display various notices. These are they!

- A health and safety poster called 'Health and Safety Law – what you should know', prominently in the practice, on general view, to ensure compliance with the Health and Safety Information for Employees Regulations 1989.

> ☑ The HSE may ask to see the practice's written health and safety policy statement. Make sure you've got one and someone knows where it is!

- A current certificate of employer's liability.
- A written Health and Safety Policy. This is a requirement for practices with five or more employees and it should be brought to their attention.
- A statement of the employer's commitment to providing a safe and healthy working environment.
- Details of safe working practices.
- Details of people responsible for health and safety throughout the workplace.

The Health and Safety Executive (HSE) is the statutory body responsible for enforcing the Health and Safety at Work Act and its inspectors have the power to inspect premises to ensure that they comply with regulations.

If there are concerns about a premises the HSE has the power to enter to inspect. If breaches of the legislation are identified, the HSE inspector can issue an improvement notice or a prohibition notice. In other words, 'fix this' or 'stop using that'. Failure to comply can result in prosecution and a hefty fine.

Other Health and Safety at Work Regulations came into force on 1 January 1993. They implement EC directives and update existing law.

They cover:

- general health and safety management
- work equipment safety
- manual handling of loads
- workplace conditions
- personal protective equipment
- display screen equipment.

So, to start, check the following:

- Does the premises comply with applicable local building codes and regulations?
- Do you have adequate public liability insurance to cover your premises?
- Is there a certificate of public liability insurance on display?

DUTIES TO STAFF

These are the practice's duties as an employer. Employers must ensure, as far as is practicable, the safety and welfare at work of all employees. This duty extends to patients and any other individuals who may be legitimately on the premises.

All systems of work must be safe and without risk to health. This applies to all equipment used within the place of work. Equipment must be regularly maintained, serviced and renewed. Safe systems of work must be in place for all persons.

You must:

- provide a written policy statement on health and safety if you employ five or more staff.
- provide and maintain safe equipment, appliances and systems of work.
- assess all equipment and systems of work for risk.
- initiate safe systems of work.
- maintain the place of work, including the means of entrance and exit, in a safe condition.
- provide a working environment for employees that is safe, without risk to health and with adequate facilities and arrangements for their welfare at work.

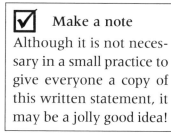

☑ Make a note
Although it is not necessary in a small practice to give everyone a copy of this written statement, it may be a jolly good idea!

- provide the necessary instruction, training and supervision to ensure health and safety.
- arrange safe disposal of waste.
- ensure that dangerous or potentially harmful substances or articles are handled and stored safely.

Practices that employ five or more staff must prepare a written statement of their policy 'with respect to health and safety' of its employees. This must include details of the organisation and arrangements for carrying out this policy and the immediate action required by staff in respect of any accidents that may occur.

Health and safety statements usually consist of three parts:

- a statement of intent which is a declaration of the employer's commitment to providing a safe and healthy workplace and environment

- details of responsibilities for health and safety throughout the workplace
- details of safe systems of work and safe working practices for all work activities.

The statement should also include the practice's policy on violence, infection control and first-aid arrangements.

DUTIES TO STAFF CHECKLIST

There's not a lot of options here. It's just got to be done.

	Done	Doing it	Who by?	When?
• Does the practice understand the duties to staff?				
• Does the practice undertake a risk assessment of the potential hazards of the practice?				
• Does the practice review the materials used in the practice?				
• Is the practice satisfied that all systems are safe and without risk to health?				
• Does a practice with more than five staff provide a written policy statement on health and safety?				
• Does the practice maintain the place of work in a safe condition?				
• Does the practice provide the necessary instruction, training and supervision to ensure health and safety?				
• If applicable does the practice arrange the safe disposal of waste?				
• Are potentially harmful substances handled and stored safely?				
• Does the practice strongly advise all staff to be immunised against diphtheria, tetanus, whooping cough, TB, rubella and hepatitis B?				

PREMISES

So far as is reasonably practicable, any place of work under the practice's control must ensure that the building is maintained in a safe condition without risks to health. There must be a safe means of entrance and exit for staff and patients.

If the practice occupies a rented building or a health centre under the control of a PCT you must do what is reasonable, but you have a duty to maintain what the lease requires you to do, and you should notify the landlord of anything that should be maintained by him, e.g. loose guttering.

If you have made the necessary notification, be sure it is in writing (and you have kept a copy). You would be in a much better position if an accident occurred. If you take out a lease, have your lawyer take a good look at it to make sure that yours and the landlord's maintenance responsibilities are clearly stated in the lease.

Remember, even if you do not own premises, you will continue to be held responsible for hazards such as slippery floors and unsafe electrical flex.

Health and safety at work legislation also states that, as far as reasonably practicable, the employer must provide and maintain a working environment for employees, which is without risk to health and with adequate provision for their general welfare.

☢ The wording appears to apply to more than just the physical environment of the employee. The practice would be well advised to consider whether there is an adequate rest room, refreshment facilities and toilet and washing arrangements, etc. The extent to which this can be done depends on the practice's resources.

Alterations to existing buildings and new premises building should take account of health and safety, and security aspects of practice. There should be wide doorways, grab rails, ramps and as few steps as possible to accommodate the elderly and infirm, children and people in wheelchairs and to meet disabled person legislation (*see* later).

The law makes provision for staff representatives and safety committees. If you have staff in a union that you recognise and if two or more safety representatives ask for a safety committee, the employer must establish one.

Premises checklist

	Yes	No	Fix it	By when?	Who?
• Do the practice principals understand who has responsibility for maintaining the building?					
• Is the building maintained in a safe condition without a risk to health?					
• Do the premises comply with applicable building codes and regulations?					
• Is there a safe means of entrance and exit for staff?					
• Are there designated and clearly marked fire exits and fire extinguishers?					
• Is adequate lighting and ventilation provided in all areas?					
• Is there disabled access to the premises?					
• Are there adequate toilet facilities?					
• Is a non-smoking policy in place and enforced?					
• Are there adequate rest and changing areas for staff?					
• Is adequate, comfortable seating available?					
• Is the reception/waiting area visible to the receptionist?					
• Do reception and examination areas assure patients of privacy during interviews, examinations and treatment?					

DUTIES TO OTHER USERS OF PRACTICE PREMISES

The primary purpose of the Health and Safety at Work Act 1974 is to ensure the safety of employees but it also applies to all persons who enter the premises – all visitors, patients and tradespersons such as postmen, window cleaners, builders, electricians, tax inspectors and even your mother-in-law . . .

> ☢ The Act imposes a duty on the practice partners as 'controller' of the premises, to ensure the safety of legitimate visitors.

The law requires that the practice is conducted in such a way as to ensure, as far as reasonably practicable, that all persons not in their employment are not exposed to risks to their health and safety when they visit.

The Act links up with the Disability Discrimination Act 1995 (*see* later) and the Occupier's Liability Act of 1957, which is too labarinthyne to go into in detail but suffice to say, you should remove any obvious hazards, with particular regard to the safety of the elderly, infirm and disabled.

The key difference between this duty and the practice's own staff is that staff should have a written safety policy and have instruction and supervision on safety matters and specific arrangements should be made for their health, safety and welfare.

EMPLOYER'S LIABILITY

The Employer's Liability (Compulsory Insurance) Act 1969 requires an employer to have adequate insurance and to display a certificate to that effect. New regulations came in during 1999 to supplement the 1969 regulations, which remain in force.

> Responsibilities lie with the practice owner(s) and with the staff. Employers and employees should co-operate to provide a safe place of work. Employees should take reasonable care of their own health and safety.

Employers must have £5 million of cover and employers will be required to keep certificates of insurance for **40** years. Yes, 40 years.

Practice premises must also be covered by adequate public liability insurance and a certificate to that effect must be displayed.

The Occupier's Liability Acts 1957 and 1984 regulate the duty which an occupier of premises owes to his or her visitors in respect of damages due to the state of the premises or to things which have been done to them or which have not been done to them. Generally this means that premises must have adequate lighting, safe stairways and all that sort of commonsense stuff.

Staff are responsible for:

* health and safety with regard to themselves, their colleagues and their patients
* abiding by health and safety rules of the practice
* reporting anything which could compromise health and safety to the person in charge.

Every employee is under a duty not to interfere intentionally or recklessly with, or misuse anything provided for the purposes of, health, safety and welfare. This protects appliances and arrangements to ensure people's safety, such as fire escapes, fire extinguishers and hazard warning notices. This could be extended to include interference with anything provided for welfare purposes, such as cloakroom and refreshment facilities.

ENFORCEMENT

The Act covers all places of employment and the Health and Safety Executive (HSE) therefore has the right to inspect Practices. The HSE is divided into areas and each has a team of inspectors.

Inspectors have a warrant of appointment that states their extensive powers and the practice manager must be bold enough to ask to see this for identification.

> ✍ **Make a note**
> Inspectors normally give notice of their visits and ring to make an appointment. Occasionally a visit may be reactive to a complaint from an employee or a patient, or they may make an unannounced call simply because it fits conveniently into a schedule for visits to other premises!

Inspectors have the right to enter any premises and enforce the Act. They do not have to seek permission or give notice of entry. They may, however, only enter at a 'reasonable time'.

During a visit, an inspector can interview and take written statements from anyone who may have relevant information, including patients as well as staff. The inspector may want information or to establish the facts about an accident or evidence for legal proceedings.

> ☢ Any information will normally be treated as confidential. The information, however, may be disclosed, subsequently, if a prosecution is brought against the employer.

WHAT ARE THE INSPECTORS LOOKING FOR?

- A statement of general policy on health and safety, and instructions on safety procedures if the practice has more than five staff.
- Compliance with the requirement to carry out a risk assessment under the Management of Health and Safety at Work Regulations 1999.
- Evidence of a good general approach to management of health and safety, specifically:
  - a record of accidents
  - electrical equipment which is in safe working order and properly maintained
  - normal standards of toilet and washing facilities
  - hot and cold running water (inspectors may also recommend that wrist-operated taps should be fitted in rooms used for examinations and treatment of patients)
  - condition of the heating plant
  - storage of drugs if appropriate
  - condition of sterilisers
  - standards of heating and lighting.

IMPROVEMENT AND PROHIBITION NOTICES

After completing an inspection, the inspector will usually talk to the person in administrative charge of the building about any improvements to safety procedures and standards that may be required. If they are minor, the inspector will simply ask for them to be put right.

If there is something more serious, the inspector may write formally or issue a written notice requiring things to be remedied. This is called an **improvement notice**. It will specify a time limit of not less than 21 days within which the improvement must be made. The inspector must inform staff as well as the practice owner of the service of the notice.

A prosecution alleging a specific breach of a statutory provision may also be brought.

If there is a serious risk to health and safety, an inspector may issue a **prohibition notice** forbidding the offending work activity.

> The inspector should also advise you of the procedure for appeal against the provisions of the notice – very comforting!

If the position is very grave, the notice will take immediate effect and work must stop at once. Otherwise a deferred prohibition notice may be issued stopping the work after a specified time.

Improvement and prohibition notices are served both on the person carrying out or in control of the work in question and normally on the practice owner.

A person on whom notice is served may appeal to an employment tribunal within 21 days of the notice being served. An improvement notice is suspended pending the outcome but a prohibition notice remains in force until the appeal is determined. When complied with, notices cease.

Don't mess with inspectors!

They can:

* issue an improvement notice which specifies what legal requirements are being broken, what action is required to put matters right and the period of time allowed
* issue a prohibition notice if there is a risk of serious personal injury
* seize, render harmless or destroy any substance or article considered to be the cause of imminent danger or serious personal injury

> Failure to comply with a prohibition notice can result in a jury trial and imprisonment for up to two years.

* prosecute any person contravening a relevant statutory provision, either instead of or in addition to serving a notice. Conviction can result in a fine of up to £20 000 for some offences.

Because the Health and Safety at Work Act is a criminal statute, contravention of its provisions may lead to a fine or imprisonment.

Both the employer and the staff may be liable for prosecution. Alongside the criminal prosecution, an employee could sue an employer for damages on the basis of employers' liability law, or simply for negligence. Wow!

Time for a cuppa. or something stronger . . .

FIRST AID AND COLLAPSE ROUTINE

This may be necessary if you have just read the health and safety information in the previous section!

Under the Health and Safety (First Aid) Regulations 1981 all employers must make adequate first aid provisions. Ideally, a first aid person should be nominated and all employees should know where the first aid box is kept.

All staff members (including the GPs and nurses!) should be trained, up-to-date, in cardiopulmonary resuscitation and prepared to deal with any emergency. Up-to-date is the key phrase here!

Apart from any legislative requirements, failure to be able to manage an emergency (cardiac arrest, diabetic collapse, epileptic fit, etc.) will reflect badly on the GP and the practice. (Probably the understatement of the book – Ed.)

A first aid box should be provided and it should contain:

- a guidance card on resuscitation
- individually wrapped sterile adhesive dressings (various sizes)
- individually wrapped triangular bandages
- medium-sized individually wrapped sterile un-medicated wound dressings (approximately 10 cm × 10 cm)
- large sterile individually wrapped un-medicated wound dressings
- other wound dressings
- safety pins
- sterile eye pads and attachments.

> ✍ First aid boxes should not contain medication of any kind.

FIRE SAFETY

The Fire Precautions (Workplace) Regulations 1997 require the employer to assess what fire precautions are needed by carrying out a fire risk assessment under the Management of Health and Safety at Work Regulations 1999.

> ✍ If you are in a big practice remember that in buildings with more than 20 employees or more than 10 staff working on floors other than the ground floor, the owner of the premises is required to obtain a certificate from the local fire authority regulating the means of escape and marking fire exits.

Employers are required to ensure that proper consideration has been given to fire prevention. The regulations require an employer to ensure that:

- emergency routes and exits are kept clear of obstructions
- they should lead directly to a place of safety
- they should be clearly indicated
- fire detection devices and fire fighting equipment should be in good working order and regularly checked
- a system should be in place ensuring that, in the event of a fire, the number of people in the practice at that time can be identified.

Premises should be equipped with properly maintained alarms and the employees should be familiar with the means of escape and the routine to be followed in the event of a fire. There should be emergency lighting as necessary. Local fire inspectors will ensure that these requirements are complied with.

Make sure that:

- a fire can be detected in a reasonable time and people warned
- automatic fire detection is considered
- people in the building can get out safely
- there is adequate fire fighting equipment available
- a fire extinguisher is provided for each 200 square metres of floor space with a minimum of one per floor
- all employees know what to do in the event of a fire
- fire equipment is regularly checked and maintained.

Emergency routes and exits should:

- be kept free of obstruction at all times
- lead directly to a place of safety
- be appropriately and clearly indicated
- have emergency lighting if required
- open in the direction of escape and in an easy and immediate action.

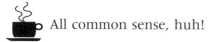 All common sense, huh!

FIRE CHECKLIST

	Yes	No	Will be sorted	By when?	Who by?
• Is all appropriate fire fighting equipment available?					
• Is fire fighting equipment serviced regularly?					
• Are escape routes and exits clear and appropriately signed?					
• Are extinguishers appropriately signed?					
• Are fire and smoke alarms installed, maintained and tested regularly?					
• Are practice staff trained to respond to fire?					
• Is fire drill practised regularly?					
• Is a fire drill notice displayed in the practice?					
• Do staff have written protocols about fire procedures?					

ELECTRICITY REGULATIONS

This time it is the Electricity at Work Regulations 1989. They are concerned with the safety of both the fixed supply to the premises and any moveable (portable) appliances.

> ✍ **Make a note**
>
> If someone receives a shock or worse, compliance with legislation in respect of inspection and testing would be vital to your defence.

Electrical equipment must be in good working order at all times. All earthed equipment and most leads and plugs connected to equipment should have an occasional combined inspection and test by an appropriately trained person to identify any faults which may not be found by a visual check.

The Health and Safety Executive (them again) has suggested intervals of up to five years in low risk environments depending on the type of equipment used.

There are contract electricians who will provide this type of service. They put little stickers on things to show they've tested them. They'll even remember when they last checked your equipment and come round and do it again – when the time (and the price!) is right.

If it is time for ☕ make sure that the electric kettle is safe!

	Yes	No	Will be sorted	By when?	By whom?
• Have you got a programme for ensuring electrical equipment is safe at all times?					
• Is electrical equipment installed by appropriate contractors?					
• Is all electrical equipment earthed?					
• Is all electrical equipment provided with fuses of the correct amperage?					
• Is electrical equipment maintained regularly and a record kept?					
• Is electrical wiring checked regularly to inspect for cable or plug damage?					
• Are staff vigilant to the possibility of equipment overheating and aware to whom such problems should be reported?					

COSHH REGULATIONS

Maybe you don't use any hazardous substances – breathe a sigh of relief. Skip this and make a brew!

✎ The regulations apply to most hazardous substances except those covered by their own legislation, such as asbestos, lead and materials producing ionising radiations.

The Control of Substances Hazardous to Health Regulations 1999 (COSHH) set out the legal framework for the management of health risks from the exposure to hazardous substances used at work.

They aim to prevent occupational ill-health by encouraging employers to assess and prevent or control risks from exposure to hazardous substances in a systematic and practical way.

The regulations set out the measures that employers and employees have to take. Failure to comply exposes people to risk and constitutes an offence under health and safety at work legislation.

Hazardous substances include those labelled as dangerous (toxic, harmful, irritant or corrosive).

Practices may have to be careful about certain cleaning fluids, phenolics, formaldehyde or glutaraldehyde used as chemical disinfectants and clinical waste, either in medicine or in related specialities.

All employers should consider how COSHH applies to their employees and working environment. For most practices, compliance should be very straightforward.

This is what you do:

- Identify hazardous substances.
- Assess the risk to health and what precautions are required.
- Record the precautions in writing.
- Introduce measures to prevent or control exposure.
- Ensure that control measures are used.
- Inform and instruct employees about risks and precautions to be taken.

Simple!

WASTE DISPOSAL

Waste disposal depends on
what you have to dispose
of, which in turn reflects
the sort of practice that is
carried out.

> ✏️ Waste disposal basic requirements:
> - Have a written practice waste disposal
>   policy.
> - Arrange for safe transportation and col-
>   lection of waste and safe disposal in
>   accordance with legislation.
> - If in doubt, regard waste as clinical.

The Environmental Pro-
tection Act 1990 places a duty of care to sort waste, store it safely in a
suitable container and arrange for its safe disposal.

There is a requirement to document disposal routes (Environmental
Protection (Duty of Care) Regulations 1991). Depending on the activities
conducted in the practice, waste must be segregated into clinical, non-
clinical, special waste and sharps.

Non-clinical waste is material such as paper, plastic, old lottery tickets, etc.
Clinical waste is contaminated by blood or other body fluids. If in doubt,
classify the waste as clinical and dispose of it accordingly.

Clinical waste must be transported in UN-approved rigid containers. Yes,
that is UN as in United Nations (Carriage of Dangerous Goods (Classification,
Packaging and Labelling) and Use of Transportable Pressure Receptacles
Regulations 1996). Sharps must be contained in sealable UN-type approved
'sharps' containers to BS 7320.

Clinical waste and sharps must be collected by authorised persons and
documentation of the waste content provided and records of transfer held by
both parties. Transfer notes may cover repeated transfers up to one year. You
must keep the documentation for two years – and then dispose of it as non-
clinical waste about clinical waste – clear?

Special waste is prescribed medicines and other waste classified as
irritant, harmful, toxic, carcinogenic or corrosive. You probably haven't
got any. If you have, get a copy of the Special Waste Regulations 1996.
Gripping stuff!

Waste disposal checklist

	Yes	No	Will be sorted	By whom?	By when?
• Are you aware of the different types of waste and the requirements for the correct disposal of each?					
• Is practice waste correctly categorised, stored and disposed of?					
• Is clinical waste stored in appropriate containers?					
• Are staff trained in its disposal?					
• Do staff only handle clinical waste when using heavy duty rubber gloves?					
• Are systems in place for the correct transfer of waste?					
• Is waste collected by an authorised person?					
• Has the practice checked the certificate of registration of the waste remover?					
• When clinical waste is removed, is a signature obtained by the practice?					
• Are transfer notes kept for two years?					
• Are 'sharps' sealed in UN-type approved containers?					
• Does the practice ever create special waste?					

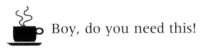 Boy, do you need this!

Computers

A computer screen is becoming as common as a stethoscope. Indeed, the new GMS contract is all but inoperable without computers, technology and software. There's no hiding place, the practice is just going to have to get this right.

Try and get the checklist ticked off, done and dusted. First, here are four basic points:

• For regular VDU users there are responsibilities under the Health and Safety (Display Screen Equipment) Regulations 1992, to assess the workplace and to take steps to reduce any identified risks.

- Employees should be trained to use their workstation correctly in order to avoid health problems.
- The type of training and the date provided should be recorded.
- Responsibilities under data protection and other legislation regarding the rights of patients concerning confidentiality and access to clinical records. (We've already looked at Data Protection – flick back to pages 91–4.)

There's not a lot else to say, so, brace yourself for the checklist!

	Yes	No	On someone's to do list	By whom?	By when?
• Who regularly uses Display Screen Equipment (DSE)?					
• Do computer users include those people continuously at a screen for longer than one hour at a time, using a PC every day or needing to use a PC to do the job?					
• Have the workstations been assessed?					
• Have the workstations been upgraded or changed to rectify any problems with the workstation set-up identified at risk management?					
• Are free eyesight tests regularly offered to all DSE users?					
• Are employees aware that they should report any discomfort in working with DSE?					
• Are computer users instructed and trained in their use?					
• Are records kept of workstation assessments, eyesight tests and results and are corrective appliances offered and details of information and training provided?					
• Do images on screen flicker or jump?					
• Can the user adjust the brightness and contrast controls on the PC? Is instruction required to enable them to do this?					

	Yes	No	On someone's to do list	By whom?	By when?

- Can the user tilt or swivel the screen to avoid glare and allow maintenance of a comfortable posture?
- Is the screen clean and are cleaning materials available?
- Is the keyboard tiltable and separate from the screen (apart from wire connections) allowing the user to adjust the keyboard to suit their needs?
- Does the keyboard have a matt surface to avoid reflective glare?
- Is there sufficient space in front of the keyboard to allow users to rest their wrists whilst keying in?
- Is a wrist rest required and, if so, has it been supplied?
- Is a mouse necessary and has a mouse mat been supplied?
- Is the work area provided adequate to accommodate the range of tasks performed?
- Can unessential items be relocated?
- Is a document holder required and has one been provided?
- Does the work chair allow the user to obtain a comfortable posture and is the seat adjustable for height, lumbar support and tilt?
- Does the user require a footrest (do the feet reach the floor when sitting) and if so has one been provided?

Environment
- Do the user's legs fit comfortably under the work surface?
- Does the workstation allow a comfortable posture for the user?
- Is lighting appropriate for the tasks being undertaken?

	Yes	No	On someone's to do list	By whom?	By when?

Environment (cont.)

- Is there glare or reflection from the screen and, if so, have steps been taken to control it using window blinds, lighting adjustment or an antiglare screen?
- Is noise a problem and, if so, what is proposed for its reduction?
- Are temperature and humidity levels appropriate?

Task design and software

- Is the task designed to ensure variety, allowing the user to take regular breaks to undertake other tasks?
- Can users take breaks from the screen at their own discretion?
- Are users involved in the planning, design and implementation of tasks?
- Does the software used enable users to complete tasks efficiently without presenting unnecessary problems or stress?
- Are users fully trained to operate the software used and have further training requirements been identified?
- Does the software provide on-line help and feedback to the user (e.g. as error messages, etc.)
- Is there a system of task checking (whereby managers can check the amount of work being generated by employees) and are employees aware of this?

MANUAL HANDLING

It would be jolly awkward for a practice to fall foul of these regulations: the Manual Handling Operations Regulations 1992.

They place responsibilities on both the employer and employee to ensure that handling is reduced to a minimum and mechanical aids are used wherever possible.

Training in handling should be given to all staff and employees must use equipment where it is provided. The employer must assess the risks taking into account the loads involved, the environment in which the handling takes place and the individual capacity for carrying out the task.

It would be the height of embarrassment if you hurt your own back – be careful!

PROTECTIVE CLOTHING

The Personal Protective Equipment (PPE) at Work Regulations 1992 require an employer to provide protective clothing where it is necessary to ensure safe systems at work. PPE made or sold in the UK must carry the CE marking and necessary information. Surgery clothing must be of a material that can be washed at a temperature of 65°C. Eye and hand protection should be provided and the employer must ensure that it is used by the employee if it is required.

☢ Medical gloves for single use (to BS EN 455) should be worn for relevant clinical procedures.

Care should be taken when choosing latex gloves, as latex is covered by the COSHH Regulations. So there should be no cutting corners with cheap gloves, no matter how persuasive the rep may be.

Further advice is contained in the Medical Devices Agency's (now the Medicines and Healthcare Regulation Agency [MHRA]) publication *Latex Sensitisation in the Health Care Setting (use of latex gloves) (DB 9601)*.

REPORTING OF INJURIES, DISEASES AND DANGEROUS OCCURRENCES

Also known as RIDDOR (love that acronym!), the Reporting of Injuries, Diseases and Dangerous Occurrences Regulations 1995, impose duties on employers to notify the Health & Safety Executive (HSE) of accidents causing death or major injury in the workplace.

They impose a statutory duty on all employers to keep a record of accidents occurring on their premises and to notify the HSE of certain serious accidents.

The employer is responsible for reporting any accident or dangerous occurrence and may be responsible for reporting a case of an occupational disease. It is wise to assume that you should report the latter.

> ☢ All accidents must be recorded in a practice accident book.
>
> Major accidents must be reported to the HSE immediately by telephone and within 10 days on form F2508.

Any notifiable accident must be directly notified to the local office of the HSE by telephone. Keep a written record of the call including the name of the person receiving it and details of the accident, occurrence or disease. A written report should be sent to the HSE within 10 days.

Notifiable dangerous occurrences are also defined in the Regulations and include explosion, electrical short circuit or overload attended by fire or explosion, which resulted in stoppage of plant for more than 24 hours. Plant? That's for factories isn't it? Well, yes and no; accidents involving explosion of an autoclave could be notifiable.

Employers must make and keep a record of all reported injuries and dangerous occurrences. Under the regulations certain types of diseases must also be reported when a person is carrying out work in a GP surgery, such as TB.

✍ What do you report? Here's a list of the basics:

- Record any accidents in the practice accident book.
- If a major accident occurs in the practice the HSE must be notified immediately by telephone and within 10 days on form F2508.
- Dangerous occurrences must be reported, i.e. if something happens which does not result in an injury but could have done so.
- If an accident happens to an employee in your practice and causes that employee to be absent for three days or more, the HSE must be notified.
- If an employee suffers from a reportable work-related disease, the HSE must be informed.

If an accident occurs you must record:

- date and time of the accident
- name and occupation of the injured party
- nature of the injury
- where it occurred
- name and address of witnesses and any other relevant information.

WRITTEN RECORDS OF RIDDOR (SOUNDS LIKE SOMETHING FROM LORD OF THE RINGS!)

A record must be kept of all notifiable accidents and dangerous occurrences, so that the employer can monitor these and identify any preventive action that should be taken. Failure to do so could lead to a fine of up to £5000.

Major accidents that need to be reported include:

 Incidentally . . .
If the accident happens to a GP and they are 'the employer', that is, a practice principal, they need not report an accident to him or herself. See, nobody loves you. Not even the Health and Safety Executive.

- fractures of the skull, spine or pelvis
- fracture of any bone in the arm or leg (except in the wrist, hand, ankle or foot)
- amputation of a hand or foot

- dislocation of the shoulder, hip, knee or spine
- loss of sight in an eye
- loss of consciousness through lack of oxygen
- any other injury resulting in a person being admitted to hospital as an inpatient for more than 24 hours, unless detained only for observation.

Notifiable dangerous occurrences include:

- explosion
- electrical short circuit.

SAFETY SIGNS

If you're into details about safety signs, try the Health and Safety Executive. Their website is at: www.hse.gov.uk. However, here are the basics.

The Health and Safety (Safety Signs and Signals) Regulations 1996 apply to all workplaces and place a duty on employers to use a safety sign wherever a hazard exists that cannot be adequately controlled by any other means.

☑ **Checklist**
- All safety signs should carry a pictogram.
- Fire fighting equipment and unobstructed fire escape routes must be adequately sign-posted and contain information on assembly points.
- A safety sign must be displayed locating the first aid facilities and identifying the designated person.

You should have a minimum of the following signs within the practice:
- **Fire safety signs:** these must provide safety information on escape routes, emergency exits, location of fire fighting equipment and a means of giving warning in the event of fire.
- **First aid:** where first aid facilities are located and the designated person.

This means that, when everything else has been done to remove the hazard, safety signs should be used to reduce the risk further. Fire safety signs are within the Regulations and include information on emergency exits, escape routes and the identification of fire fighting equipment.

VENTILATION

The Workplace (Health Safety and Welfare) Regulations 1992 require enclosed workplaces to be ventilated with sufficient fresh or purified air.

This is what the combined brains of the health and safety guru community has dreamed up. Doesn't seem too difficult does it?

• Windows must be of reasonable size and able to be opened.
• Any air supply must be from a clean source.
• Sufficient air movement must be available.

RADIATION HAZARDS

If you have the facilities to do x-rays then there are another load of regulations to comply with.

In a word: the Ionising Radiations Regulations 1999, which revoke the 1985 regulations of the same name. The Ionising Radiation (Medical Exposure) Regulations 2000 revoke the Ionising Radiation (POPUMET) Regulations 1988.

It will come as no surprise that the Ionising Radiation (Medical Exposure) Regulations 2000 place duties on employers and practitioners/operators of radiation equipment:

• The employer shall ensure that written protocols are in place for every type of standard radiological practice for each piece of equipment.

In order to comply with the regulations:

• Notify the local Health and Safety Executive of radiation usage in the practice.
• Decide if a Radiation Protection Adviser (RPA) is required.
• Appoint a Radiation Protection Supervisor.
• Ensure that equipment meets required standards of radiation safety.
• Provide local rules, which must include the name of the RPS, a description of the controlled area and any special provisions of a local nature.
• A radiation safety assessment must be carried out every three years by a 'competent authority'. This will either be the National Radiological Protection Board or a local medical physics department.

- All equipment must meet all standards as recommended in 1994 guide-lines and must be serviced and maintained according to the manufacturer's specifications.
- Personal monitoring for staff by a dose meter may be required according to the number of x-rays taken per week.
- Staff must be appropriately trained.
- Local rules must include a contingency plan to specify what needs to be done following equipment malfunction.

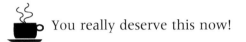 You really deserve this now!

HEALTH AND SAFETY 2

From 1 October 2004, the Disability Discrimination Act applied to small employers (not those less than 5 feet tall, those with fewer than 15 staff).

☑ **Tip**

Look at the website www.disability.gov.uk – lots of help there.

The legislation has profound implications for all healthcare premises. Many practices employ more than 15 staff, so some of this will not be new. However, the legislation now applies to everyone – so read on.

Effectively the Act means that you must be careful not to discriminate against disabled employees or job applicants because of their disability and you may have to consider making reasonable adjustments to your workplace to accommodate them.

So what is a reasonable adjustment? Under the Act you only need to make changes that are 'reasonable'. There are no set rules. Different people, patients and organisations have different needs. Some organisations can afford to do more than others. It is about practicality and availability of resources.

Here are some things that might be regarded as 'reasonable':

- rearranging furniture so that it is not an obstacle course for the disabled
- rearranging duties to accommodate a disabled employee
- allowing someone to work more flexible hours
- allowing someone time off for rehabilitation or treatment
- making arrangements for information handling for a blind person
- providing equipment for a hearing-impaired person.

☢ If someone thinks you have discriminated against someone, you can be taken to a tribunal and compensation could be awarded.

> 🖎 If you need information about any aspect of the legislation, contact the Department for Work and Pensions on 0845 124 9841 or email DDAinfopack@meads-ltd.co.uk.

Clearly what can be done will depend on the individual circumstances, the design of the premises and the resources available to the practice.

The disability legislation does not simply apply to employees. There are a load of duties already in place for you as a service provider under the Disability Discrimination Act.

You cannot refuse to treat a disabled patient or provide a lower standard of service to a disabled person because of their disability.

You should make reasonable changes to the way that you provide your service so that your disabled patients do not suffer discrimination. You should, for example, adjust any natural barriers that may prevent disabled people using your service.

The changes that you would need to make are **only those that are reasonable**. It would not be reasonable for a medical practice with (say) one or two GPs to make major structural changes to the premises at huge cost. You must consider what is practicable and what resources are available.

The law will not require you to make changes that are impractical or beyond your means.

In any case you should consider:

- ensuring that the premises are well lit
- ensuring that clear signs are provided
- ensuring the seating is appropriate for disabled patients, i.e. not too low or inaccessible
- using ramps and handrails at the entrance to a building
- ensuring that door handles are of an 'easy-grip' variety

> ☑ The Disability Rights Commission, an independent body, publishes *A Practical Guide for Small Businesses*, which is free. Alternatively, visit the DRC website at www.drc-gb.org.

- lowering part or all of the reception desk to make it more accessible for people who use wheelchairs
- using colour contrast to ensure that entrances and exits are easier to use
- seeing disabled patients on the ground floor if your surgery is on two levels.

Decisions to modify the surgery premises will depend on your individual situation and the disabled patients that you have.

Be sure to incorporate disabled-friendly facilities in any new building or refurbishments that you might be making. Remember, too, that such modifications will also help the elderly who, though not actually disabled, may appreciate easier access, as would patients with children, patients with heavy shopping bags or the friends and families of disabled patients.

> ☺ If you have some disabled patients, why not ask their views about the surgery and discuss with them what can be done.

UNDERSTANDING DISABILITY: FACT SHEET PUBLISHED BY DISABILITY.GOV.UK

The fact sheet points out that there are 10 000 000 disabled people covered by the legislation with wide-ranging impairments. Review your premises to provide good access and service to patients.

This chart is a quick checklist, modified from the leaflet:

Type of impairment	Accessibility issue	Customer service value
Mobility	• Width of doorways and aisles – consider width required for wheelchair access • Height of counters and handles • Evenness of flooring inside and outside the premises • Accessibility of WC facilities	• Ensure suitable seating which is easily accessible • Sit down to talk to wheelchair users so they do not need to crane their neck to see you • Do not lean on the wheelchair. It is part of their personal space
Sight	• Colour contrast on signs, between floors, walls, ceilings and doors • Literature and signage • Clutter and hazards – keep floors clear	• Identify yourself when speaking to a blind person • Stand still so a partially sighted patient can focus on you • If guiding someone allow them to hold your arm rather than vice versa • Do not move away without telling them
Hearing	• Write down messages if necessary • Add additional aids such as hearing loops • Have visual and audible alarm systems	• Maintain eye contact with lip-reading patients • Speak normally, keep hands away from mouth • Minimise background noise
Speech	• Consider disability awareness training to help staff communicate effectively • Clear signage and labelling	• Speak slowly and clearly • Be patient and listen. Do not speak for the patient • If you do not understand, ask them to repeat themselves • If possible, ask questions with yes or no answers
Learning disabilities	• Signage, clear and concise • Plain English with pictures and images	• Be patient and listen • Ask the person to repeat themselves • Speak clearly and use pictures and symbols

Accessibility to the premises

Checkpoint	Practical suggestions
Approaching and entering	
Can disabled people park nearby?	• Disabled parking bays? • Give information or advice about parking
Is the entrance easy to find?	• Make the door a different colour from adjacent windows • Make the name and number clearly visible. Signs perpendicular to the building may be useful
Is the entrance wide enough for all users?	• Consider width for wheelchair users • If doorway cannot be widened, install doorbell • Have glass panels in front door to see who is outside
Is the front door at street level?	• Install permanent or temporary ramp alongside steps • Provide alternative entrance accessible for all users • Speak to local council about street adjustments
Is door easy to open?	• Place door handle at accessible height for wheelchair users • Use easy-grip handle • Install magnetic device that holds doors open • Consider low-energy automatic door opener
Moving around	
Is it easy to get round premises?	• Ensure doormats are flush with floor and avoid bristle matting • Remove clutter, eliminate slippery floors • Put handrails on each side of stairs. Consider ramp or lift
Signage	• Keep simple, short and clear • Have good contrast with background, e.g. black on white • Use visual or pictorial symbols in addition to words
Is lighting good?	• Keep windows, lamps and blinds clean • Avoid glare • Light faces from in front rather than behind • Use extra lighting to highlight internal steps and safety hazards
Are floors, walls, ceilings and doors easily distinguishable?	• Use matt paint in contrasting colours or different tones
Is the alarm system and procedure effective?	• Supplement audible alarms with visual alarms • Ensure staff know how to assist disabled people in emergency
Using facilities	
Are your staff skilled in handling disabled patients?	• Allow more time • Talk to the disabled person, not to the companion • Have notepads for exchanging notes • Consider disability awareness training
Can all patients access services?	• General review of access in practice and if possible have a consulting room on the same level as the entrance/waiting area
Seating	• Use flexible seating, of different heights with and without armrests • Have space by chair(s) for a wheelchair to pull up alongside a seated companion
Toilet facilities	• Adequate disabled access to toilet • Wheelchair accessible standards including getting to and from the toilet • Ensure toilet door can be opened with appropriate device from the outside • Provide an alarm pull
Are alternative facilities available if modifications cannot be made?	• Consider providing the service in an alternative location, either by appointment or regularly • Provide an at-home service and ensure that patients are aware of it

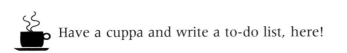 Have a cuppa and write a to-do list, here!

EMPLOYMENT ISSUES AND RISK

Employment issues are a minefield that is really a life's work and, unfortunately, outside the scope of this book – we don't have enough pages! The legislation regarding the employment of staff is complex and changes more often than David Beckham's haircut.

If your practice is a 'a sole practitioner' and you are contemplating the employment of staff you should obtain appropriate advice.

If you already have staff but perhaps you are not confident that you have done everything by the book, or if you feel that a problem might be brewing, a good place to mug-up is with these two most helpful websites:

- the Advice, Conciliation and Arbitration Service (ACAS): www. acas.org.uk
- the Department of Trade and Industry (DTI): www.dti.gov.uk.

 Get browsing . . .

RECRUITMENT AND EMPLOYMENT: SOME BASIC CONSIDERATIONS

Hiring staff of the right quality and skill level is a great talent. To get it right you must think like a recruiter. It is easy to be impressed by the wrong things! You need to have clear objectives.

For example, when recruiting a part-time receptionist, the wrong receptionist can easily cause damage to your reputation, your income and your cardiovascular system when you get cross!

New staff have to have the right talents and they have to 'fit' into the job and the practice environment.

There are three levels of 'fit' that you may want to consider:

- **Practice fit:** What kind of employee are you seeking? Are you looking for initiative, problem-solving, customer care skills or simple administrative abilities?
- **Team fit:** Would your new employee bring the right qualities and personality?
- **Role fit:** Does your potential new employee have the appropriate technical and other skills and qualifications?

How you are going to find your new employee?

First, produce a job description. For instance, for an administrative role, list the required skills and competencies. Also include working hours, details of role, required computer and communication skills and any other ancillary competencies such as book-keeping, advertising or support for clinical work.

> ☢ Avoid recruiting a friend's daughter or the next door neighbour. You may well end up with a totally inappropriate employee, an acrimonious dismissal and damage to friend or family relationships!

If you expect your new employee to make your tea and buy your Hobnobs, make it clear from the start. The employee should not be surprised by the nature or scope of their role once they have started work. Also make the salary explicit so that there are no embarrassing discussions about money at a later stage.

Decide where you will place an advertisement. It may be on local noticeboards, in the local newspaper or using an employment agency.

Read all the applications carefully. Look out for unexplained gaps in the previous employment history.

Score the applications against the skills and competencies that you seek. Make sure you don't allow bias or prejudices to creep into your

> ☢ If you do decide to interview candidates who are recommended for the role by friends or relatives, explain at the outset that you will review them using the same criteria as other interviewees. Think **very carefully** before you consider a patient for a staff role.

assessment. Take up references of potential employees if they have agreed that you may do so before interview. Many likely employees will not want you to tell their existing employer that they are looking for a new job and so will only permit the taking of a reference once you have offered the post. That's fair enough.

Plan your interview

If you are fortunate enough to have a good response and a large number of candidates who appear to meet your requirements, think about arranging the interviews in two stages, preliminary and final. If you do, you must make it clear to the applicants what you are doing.

If the GPs or nursing staff are to be involved in the interviews, they will probably be better done out of surgery hours. This makes sure the clinicians are not called away and that you can take the opportunity to show the candidate the practice and explain the details of any tasks that might be unfamiliar (for example operating an autoclave).

It also gives the opportunity for the candidate to decide whether the job is really the sort of post they are looking for. Better to have an applicant withdraw at the preliminary stage than two weeks after starting the job.

After the preliminary stage, aim to reduce the numbers to a more manageable number. Three is ideal.

What happens at the interview?

If there is an interview panel, bear in mind: there is little worse than a candidate confronted by an interview panel that hasn't planned its questions in advance!

Consider carefully who will actually conduct the interview. Should it be done by someone alone or as part of a small panel? The bigger the panel, the more complicated and sometimes clumsy the process can be.

Bear in mind, one or two people who can offer independent views may be very valuable in helping you to make your decision.

Make a list of all the key questions you want the answers to and share them out between panel members.

Once you have made your decision, make clear that any job offer is subject to satisfactory references and if you have not already done so, **always take up the references**.

☺ A panel of seven to interview someone applying for a 10-hour-a-week receptionist post would be huge overkill! But they should be seen by more than one person . . .

☑ Always check what your preferred candidate's resignation arrangements are. Will they have to work a long notice period? Does that impact on your plans?

Once you have done the checking and are satisfied that the candidate is the employee for you, telephone them to make a firm offer. It is friendly and welcoming.

Confirm the offer in writing, incorporating details of the principal elements of the post including hours and salary.

Once the new employee is in post, you need to ensure they have:

- a job description – this is not a legal obligation but very sensible best practice
- a contract of employment providing the terms and conditions of the employment.

The contract should normally have the following components:

- title of post
- key elements of role
- hours and place of employment
- holiday entitlement, types of leave and accumulation of leave
- probation period (if applicable)
- remuneration and overtime payments
- payment of bonuses (if applicable)
- illness and certification
- disciplinary procedure
- grievance procedure
- counselling
- unilateral changes.

> ☑ Make sure you do things right!
> Make proper arrangements for payment. Paying cash out of the petty cash should not be the method of choice unless clearly sanctioned by your accountant.
> Ask them to help you get proper payroll arrangements sorted.
> They may even do it for you.

The employee should be provided with a written statement of the terms and conditions within 13 weeks of the commencement of the employment.

Many of the problems that arise during the course of employing staff relate to failures of communication. Much of this can be eliminated by having a handbook that informs the staff member of the elements of the employment in more detail.

It may also contain policies referred to in the contract. Although it may seem to be 'over the top' to give a receptionist an employee's handbook, when there may only be one or two staff members, it does provide a way of ensuring that ambiguities within the professional relationship are minimised.

Here's what a handbook might contain.

A statement of your expectations of the staff member

You can use the section to describe the way in which you would expect a staff member to work, behave and manage patients. You might want to comment on the issues surrounding the acceptance of patients, any expectations you might have in terms of collecting information about them and what to do if the patient was difficult or behaved inappropriately. It is a good idea to take the opportunity to include a list of generic tasks or to make reference to the job description.

Appraisal

You should have an annual appraisal system for your staff. There may be circumstances where either you have a problem with him or her, or they have a problem with you, or their role within the practice. Providing an opportunity to review the year, to assess the progress of the practice, to identify any difficulties in its operation, to review the employee's role and to consider educational needs and opportunities for development is often very valuable and will allow you to make your practice more successful.

Absence

In small practice the absence of a staff member may have a very serious effect on the function of the practice. You may wish to try to minimise the disruption by asking the staff member:

- to let you know by (say) 9.00 a.m. if he or she is sick and cannot work
- to provide a self-certificate for the first seven days of illness
- to provide a medical certificate for longer periods of illness
- to ensure that he or she is fit to return to work before doing so
- to co-operate if you wish to make enquiries from her medical advisers to understand the reasons for the absence from work.

Maternity leave

You may wish to record details of taking time for antenatal appointments, the employee's rights in respect of returning to work after a pregnancy, payments made during maternity leave and any other information you may wish to give.

Holiday entitlements

The number of days off per year, arrangements for public holidays, etc.

Disciplinary procedures

This is a difficult area and the topic could be a book in itself. However, here is a summary.

If problems arise with a staff member and there is no documented disciplinary or grievance procedures, it will be far more difficult to take effective action to control the situation.

The procedure must be fair and equitable.

Disciplinary procedures are designed to ensure that there is fair and prompt action. The aim is to bring about improvement through guidance, training and encouragement.

Disciplinary procedure consists of four stages:

1 verbal warning
2 first written warning
3 final written warning
4 dismissal.

The level at which the procedure starts depends on the seriousness of the offence. In your booklet you may wish to describe how you will administer the disciplinary process at any given stage.

Employees have a right to appeal against any disciplinary action taken against them. The disciplinary policy notified in the contract of employment should be referred to in the handbook.

Grievance

You will want to create an environment where, if employees have a problem (grievance) with their employment, they feel able to raise it with you, so that you can attempt to deal with it quickly and satisfactorily.

The grievance policy notified in the contract may be included in the handbook.

Computer and Visual Display Unit (VDU) usage

See the section on IT to notify the employee of the conditions of use of computers.

Electronic mail

The purpose of the email is to conduct professional business.

Messages and email equipment are the property of the practice.

Spell out the fact that no emails are private and you reserve the right to access and disclose the contents of all messages created, sent or received using your email system.

Emails should be treated in the same way as all other professional communications. Emails should not contain material that may be considered offensive or disruptive. Offensive content includes, but is not confined to, obscene or harassing language or images, racial, ethnic and sexual or gender-specific comments or images that would offend someone on the basis of their religious or political beliefs, sexual orientation, national origin or age.

The occasional personal use of the email system is permitted but such messages become the property of the practice and are subject to the same conditions as other email.

Violation of the policy will result in disciplinary action up to and including termination and/or legal action if warranted.

Health and safety

Lay out the principles of health and safety. A staff member must ensure that their health and safety and that of other users of the practice are not affected by any activity that they do or do not do at work. Staff have an obligation to minimise the possibility of an accident.

If staff identify a hazardous process it should immediately be brought to the attention of their manager.

All accidents at work should immediately be reported and recorded appropriately and all staff must comply with any local safety rules.

Specific health and safety issues that should be listed include:

- Fire safety
  - fire drill
  - fire alarm
  - fire extinguishers
- First aid equipment
- Storage of materials
  - filing cabinets
  - storage cupboards.

Lifting

The booklet should advise staff that the practice of lifting and handling is based on the following six principles:

- **feet:** hip-width apart with one foot forward in the direction of travel
- **knees:** bend to gain lifting power from the leg muscles

☢ Before you lift, ensure that the area is clean and tidy. Remove any obstacles from the area that may cause a fall, slip or trip, such as trailing wires and cables, loose carpeting or items of office furniture, and get close to the load.

Assess the weight to be lifted before attempting to do so.

- **back:** straight but not necessarily vertical, to ensure that the spine and the back muscles do not take the strain of the lift
- **hands:** grasp object to be lifted by using the whole of the fingers and the palms of the hands
- **arms:** keep them as close to the body as possible, with elbows well tucked in
- **head:** chin tucked in with load facing the direction in which you intend to move.

Key points:

- think before lifting
- use mechanical aids, e.g. trolley
- push, don't pull
- obtain assistance for heavy or awkward loads
- wear sensible footwear
- avoid wearing loose clothes
- load at waist height
- make sure that you can see over the load.

Electrical equipment

Dos and don'ts.

Accidents

What to report and to whom.

COSHH

As applicable to the practice.

ISLAM IN THE WORKPLACE

Muslims now form the largest religious group in the UK.

At a time when, with respect to the religion, considerable misunderstandings and stereotypes circulate in the media and society it is crucial to make the effort to go beyond archetypal images and to understand Islam and the Muslim faith.

The population contains approximately 1.5 million Muslims and you may well employ staff with the Muslim faith.

Here are some key issues to consider:

- prayer periods
- attendance at the mosque
- fasting periods
- dress codes
- religious holidays
- food requirements and restrictions
- physical contact.

> ☢ If Muslim employees do not feel comfortable it is likely that they will seek employment elsewhere and you may lose an excellent part of the practice team.

Employment rules and regulations are complicated. Seek advice before making precipitate changes in employment arrangements. A well-motivated and committed staff will be worth its weight in gold in the smooth running of the practice.

 Make the effort.

RISK AND THE MEDIA

There are more and more stories in the media about health. Some are good and some are, well, not so good. A generation ago, medical stories were rare and virtually only about good news; lives saved, new medical developments and so on.

> ☑ If you are ever asked for an interview of any sort, always get advice from the insurer's medico-legal adviser

Increasingly, journalists are seeking opinions and interviews from healthcare professionals, clinicians and managers.

If staff in your practice are approached, out of the blue, by journalists, think: 'why'? There may be one of two reasons:

- They may be asked to contribute to an item on a particular treatment, perhaps because they are known to favour its use, or because you are in close proximity to someone else or another practice with a different view.
- They may be contacted as an expert witness, by virtue of previous broadcasting, public speaking, learned articles or reputation to comment on a particular treatment or approach to illness or disease.

> ☢ There is, of course, a third reason why your practice might be contacted for a comment or a statement – because you are at the centre of a storm about your treatment or care of a patient or there are allegations of professional misconduct.
>
> In the latter case **it is vital that you contact your insurer immediately and seek the advice of the in-house medico-legal advisers.** You may need a lot of help to keep you out of difficulties. Fortunately incidents like this are relatively rare, but anyone can fall victim of an unpleasant or unsavoury allegation. If badly handled, the damage to practice or personal reputation, professional standing or family can be incalculable.

What to do if you are approached by a journalist or asked to do a television or radio interview?

Maybe the odds are against it but, like the boy scouts, it is best to be prepared.

Many of the principles of dealing with journalists are common to all media but there are particular features associated with each form and it is worth bearing them in mind.

NEWSPAPER JOURNALISTS

> ☺ **Exercise**
>
> You have become concerned about the way in which a local chiropracter is treating back pain sufferers.
>
> Your practice has advised your patients not to consult the chiropracter and somehow this information has attracted the notice of the local newspaper.
>
> One day you arrive at the practice and, as you walk to the door, a journalist appears and starts questioning you about your reasons for believing that your treatment is better or more appropriate than at the clinic down the road.
>
> What do you do?

Journalists call it door-stepping. People find themselves ambushed and accosted by a journalist in the hope that, in the heat of the moment, they will say something that gives him a story.

If you are confronted by a journalist in this or any similar way, **do not agree to make any comments**.

However, if you refuse to speak to them, you expose yourself to the risk that the refusal will be translated into obstruction or carry the implication that you have a guilty secret to conceal.

Many people think that the best approach is to decline to comment at that time, but offering to meet the journalist at a mutually convenient time (say) later in the day. This will often be good enough and will satisfy the journalist. It will give you time to get advice and to prepare yourself to speak to them.

Journalists have a job to do like everyone else. Their manner may be inquisitive, probing, intrusive or downright aggressive, but they will be diligent because they need the story. So, how should the situation be handled?

1 **If it is a GP that is being pressed, he or she should contact their insurer.** Discuss with the medico-legal adviser how the situation should be handled. It may be that the GP can handle the interview themselves,

depending on the content and nature of the matter being discussed, or it may be that they need some help from the adviser who may, if necessary, attend the interview.

2 Be prepared. Collect your thoughts about the issue and make sure that your knowledge is sufficient. Research any information you're not sure about, so that you can answer any professional questions authoritatively.

3 Prepare a written statement covering the issues to be discussed. Give the journalist a copy of the statement. The likelihood is that they will use it as the basis for an article.

4 Stick to the facts. Don't allow yourself to be drawn into speculation. Never comment on events outside your area of expertise.

5 Be positive.

6 Beware the 'golden question'. Some journalists will have a pleasant, non-aggressive and

☢ Bear in mind that you need a patient's consent before you comment about anything that a patient may have said. In general, it is wise not to comment in any way about a patient. There are exceptions, particularly if you are acting as a patient's advocate (for example to get improved services), but in such a case it is sensible to have the patient's written consent. Do not be drawn into criticising the patient or making reference to his or her clinical or personal information in response to remarks attributed to the patient about you.

☑ Make sure that you see everything that is written in the paper or magazine about you and keep in touch with your insurer so that any concerns can be handled effectively.

amiable interview and then make an aggressive or insulting comment, catching you by surprise. They then ask the one question to which they really want the answer (do you really earn £200k a year, did you sleep with the patient, etc.) in the hope that you may be unsettled by the previous remark and they can catch you off-guard so that you answer, well, more honestly than you might have done. **Do not respond to insults.**

TELEVISION JOURNALISM

Why would they want you on the telly for an interview?
  Do you fit into any of this:

- You are an expert.
- You are commenting on a case involving another GP or practice.
- You have made an almighty cock-up and you are the 'star' of an investigative programme such as Watchdog.
- You are a clinician and explaining a technique on a purely factual basis.

It is clear that different strategies are required for different types of interview request, if you agree to do one!

If the interview is in any way contentious, you should **contact your insurer** immediately and seek advice.

For the not so tricky situations, here is some basic advice. The television journalist's watchword is preparation. Homework will usually have been done by a researcher and generally they are very good. You may be surprised by how much they seem to know about your subject. You must remember this if you agree to appear on an interview.

First time on the telly? Don't be nervous – you will be, but we felt we had to say it!

Remember the **top 10 television tips** for handling an interview of this sort:

1 **Don't do it** unless you feel sure that you are able to. However flattered you may be to have been asked, think carefully. You must **never** assume that, because you are a GP, you will either know the answers or be able to bluff it. If you aren't an expert, don't expose yourself. Remember the old saying: 'They may think you are an idiot. Don't open your mouth and prove it!'

2 **Dress appropriately:** Do not look as though you have just finished the gardening. You need credibility with your audience and therefore you need to dress in a way that is consistent with your professional status. It will be much more difficult for you if you have to overcome a 'credibility gap'. Consider the following:
   (a) **Suit:** Standard wear for the professional classes!
   (b) **Do not wear your Hawaiian shirt:** A simple plain light blue coloured shirt is best.

(c) **Tie:** Do not wear a tie with tight circles or heavy patterns – it gets the cameras excited and produces an effect called **strobing**. Avoid Mickey Mouse, something plain is what's required.

> ☑ Overall the message is to be **quietly professional** and provide the appearance that your audience would expect to see.

(d) **Thin blouses:** Be careful not to wear blouses that are very lightweight because the bright television lights may pick out the bra underneath.

(e) **Men and women:** Forget heavy jewellery. Clunky rings make men look like Del Boy and dangly earrings make women look like Mystic Meg.

3 **Don't drink beforehand:** You do not need a drink beforehand as a loosener. Sometimes, particularly with some of the public debating programmes, speakers are taken to a hospitality suite first. If they have a few drinks they are much more likely to make comments that are 'newsworthy'. If you are invited to hospitality; soft drinks only!

4 **Demeanour and presentation:** Your general appearance is important. If you look like Shrek it is hard to make you look like Jude Law or Jennifer Aniston. However, there are a number of things you can do to look your best:

(a) Find out whether you will be sitting or standing for the interview. This is important because you will need to consider different issues in terms of appearance.

(b) Go to the loo. Don't wish you had gone halfway through the interview.

(c) Look in a mirror. Make sure your hair looks right and that your tie is straight.

(d) If you are sitting:
- Sit up straight.
- As you sit down, hold the sides of your jacket at the lower edge and pull them down as you sit down. If you do not do so, you may end up with the jacket sticking up with the collar in a V-shape behind you. On a sideways shot, you can look like the Hunch-Back of Notre Dame.

(e) If you are standing, **don't slouch**.

(f) Ladies, if you are sitting on a low couch (for example on breakfast TV), you may feel uncomfortable in a short skirt. Trousers are a better bet – this is true of sofa-style conversations on a stage at a conference.

(g) Remember that studio lights are bright. If they are shining in your eyes, you may find yourself squinting during the interview. Mention it. A technician will adjust them.

(h) If you wear variable tint lenses, remember that under studio lights they will become dark and you may look like a drugs dealer. Don't wear them unless you absolutely have to.

(i) If you are nervous and your hands are shaking, keep them out of the way. Hold the side of your chair. Don't wave them about.

(j) Don't fidget, and

(k) Don't forget to **smile**. A constant serious expression can generate feelings of doubt. However, use **caution**. Do not be seen smiling at an inappropriate point in an interview. Smile only with good news, not with bad news.

5 Understand the set-up of the interview in advance. The most important (and obvious) thing to know is whether it will be live or recorded.

(a) If it is recorded, you can stop an answer if it is going wrong. Discuss it with the interviewer before you start. He or she will not mind you re-recording an answer. Indeed, they may wish to re-ask the question. Some people suggest that you should spoil a wrong answer with rude words or a silly face so that they are not used. In general there is no need to do so. You can ask the studio to see the recording but they may not be able to or have the time to do so.

(b) If the interview is live, more care is needed. If you embark on an answer and you realise that it is going wrong, try to finish it as quickly as possible. Don't dig yourself a bigger hole!

6 Don't be a smart alec. Being too clever is **very** dangerous unless you are very good at it. Don't try to outsmart the interviewer. They virtually always get the last word. They will have dealt with clever Dicks before. Avoid jokes. It is easy to offend and irritate and they hardly ever amuse.

7 When answering, look straight and unswervingly either at the interviewer or at the camera. The interviewer will tell you which is preferred. If you look down or away from the camera you are likely to imply that you are being economical with the truth. Looking straight ahead looks sincere. As someone very famous once (nearly) said, 'you will know you're successful when you can fake sincerity'. Looking straight ahead helps with that. Just watch politicians!

8 When answering questions, watch out for bear traps:

(a) Stick to what you know.

(b) Do not be drawn into areas where you have no expertise.

(c) Keep the answers specific and to the point.

(d) If you don't know, **don't guess**.

(e) Don't get into a dispute with the interviewer.

(f) Don't react to insults.

9 Don't walk out. If the interview gets tough or aggressive, or if you are struggling to answer the questions, you might want to walk out. Don't do it. Whatever the circumstances – you'll look like the loser. Interviews are usually quite short. Stick it out.

10 When all else fails you may have to take steps to protect yourself from a question that may cause you problems. It may be that the interviewer has asked you a question to which you do not know the answer but saying that you do not know does not seem appropriate. Alternatively, you may know the answer all too well but don't want to give it. In such cases, there are a number of things you can do:

(a) Ask the interviewer to repeat the question. It gives you time to think out the answer and, in any case, the interviewer will probably ask the question differently and the second attempt may be easier to answer.

(b) Look blank and ask the interviewer to rephrase the question. He or she will have to use different words then!

(c) 'This is an interesting question and some background to the answer may be helpful' allows you to talk about a related subject where you may be able to speak with more confidence without actually addressing the original question.

(d) 'I think that the question you are really asking me' enables you to re-write your own question. Interviewers are (generally) too polite to tell you that you haven't answered their question.

(e) More blatantly, you can actually politely correct the interviewer by saying, 'I think a better question would be . . .'. This needs quite a lot of skill because the interviewer will spot this as a manoeuvre and may try to bring you back to the original question.

(f) Finally, you can just ignore the question you have been asked and wander off on an answer to a vaguely related question. If you do so positively, the interviewer may genuinely believe that you believed that to be the question and will be too polite to interrupt.

Good luck!

RADIO JOURNALISM

Radio journalism has a lot in common with television journalism but there are a number of very important differences.

1 You cannot be seen and so you can dress comfortably. There is no need to wear a jacket or tie. Nobody will know.
2 It is commonly the case that, if you are being interviewed, you will not be in the same studio as the interviewer, so you will not have to contend with being watched. It is sometimes the case that, when several people are being interviewed at the same time, none of them are in the same studio. The national radio stations have access to many studios in such diverse places as municipal offices and other public buildings. With local radio stations you are more likely to be asked to go to the radio station itself.
3 As with newspaper journalists, radio journalists may have a particular question or topic where they are seeking an answer. They may be determined in respect of this particular issue and you may find that they doggedly persist with the one question, which they may ask in different ways.
4 Your secret weapon on the radio is silence. **Silence is Golden.** If you are asked a question and you are struggling to answer it, say nothing. Radio cannot cope with silences and so the interviewer will have to cut in straight away and fill the gap, either by asking the question again (it will invariably be a bit different and possibly easier) or, if you are in a different studio, by asking whether you are still on the line. Either way, it is a reprieve.

Finally, remember that you can only do your best. However good you are, you may be caught out. However careful you are with your answers, an edited answer may sound quite different.

After you have done your interview, go home, watch it, listen to it or read it, and enjoy it, learn from it.

 Then pour yourself a stiff drink and forget it! It's over. You can't change it.

The final word

Is risk management worth the effort? Think about these points:

1 If an accident occurs you may end up with a patient – or even a member of staff or you – injured. Your duty to those you treat and who work with you should encourage you to minimise that as a possibility.
2 If you are accused of negligence you may be amazed to discover how popular you are, particularly with the local press. The neighbourhood reporter will be thoroughly fed up with reporting weddings and complaints about dog mess on the pavements. A juicy story about your negligence, especially if it is a bit lascivious, will go down a storm with the *Middle Wackett Advertiser*. They will run it week after week. Believe us; a bit of risk management is well worthwhile.
3 Negligence may mean a visit to the local court, the High Court or to the GMC. Not something that you will want to do.
4 Negligence equals claims. The greater the number of claims, the higher the cost of insurance. You know how you hate having to pay increasing premiums. In the end, the level at which those premiums are set is in your hands. Furthermore, most insurers may think twice about insuring you if they suspect that you are profligate.
5 Perhaps the best reason is that you probably take a pride in what you do. There is a real buzz when the patient thanks you profusely for curing them. You really can't enjoy the patients when things go wrong. Reduce the risk. Bask in the success. Sleep at nights!

 What do you think?

CLINICAL GOVERNANCE

NEVER MIND THE WIDTH, WHAT ABOUT THE QUALITY?

In case you've recently won the lottery and have been on a beach someplace hot with no wireless and you don't already know, here are the top line important things; in fact, the Dummy's Guide to Clinical Governance. Rip it out and stick it on the fridge door with one of those funny magnet things, or stick it on the noticeboard in the office – to make it look like you know what you're talking about:

Here are the basics:

- Processes are to be put in place to integrate quality into the organisations processes – it's everybody's business.
- Quality is a lot about leadership and that leadership is to stem from clinical team level.
- Evidence-based practice, backed up by ideas and evaluated innovation, will be systematically cascaded through the NHS.

> ☢ If someone wants to blow the whistle – how easy is it for your organisation to hear it?
> How do you separate out the meddlesome from the well intended?

- Clinical risk reduction programmes introduced.
- There will be a greater openness in detecting and investigating adverse events.
- Patients will be listened to and lessons learned from their experiences.
- Poor clinical performance will be detected earlier, to protect clinicians and patients.
- Clinical governance is the key theme in professional development.
- Improvements to the quality of clinical data captured.

In short, the NHS is finding out what industry has known for years; quality is everybody's business.

OK, THAT'S THE BASICS: WHAT ELSE?

None of this is going to happen overnight. There is a lot that is good in the NHS but a lot of it isn't so good. So the idea of CG is that it is to be 'developmental'. This is the Department of Health's way of saying 'we know it's going to take time'. The Department of Health are also saying that although they know it is going to take time, that's no excuse for not doing anything.

So there are some benchmarks on the way.

One good thing (or perhaps it is not) is that the Department of Health is not being prescriptive. In other words, they are not defining the exact methods that are to be used. They are setting out a framework along with some key principles and the rest is up to you.

So, in short, here are all the important bits:

Clinical Governance is:

- everyone's business
- involves patients and service users
- ignores departmental and service boundaries and works across them
- involves everyone in developing their professional capabilities
- continuous and evolving in its quest for improvement
- finding out what works best and doing it, every time
- based on evidence
- transparent and open.

> If the NHS is serious about CG and quality, is it right to leave so much of the implementation up to the locals? Is this how Tesco does it? How can there be consistent quality in the NHS if everyone is being left to do their own thing. On the other hand, how much store is to be set against the ownership of a quality strategy? If folk don't own it, they won't do it and mean it . . .

Clinical governance is not:

- a stick to bash the docs with
- another management fad
- a 'blame' thing

- tribal
- an excuse for not doing things
- up to someone else to do
- keeping quiet about things that go wrong.

Clinical Governance recognises:

> 'A quality service is built by: being open about the strengths and weaknesses of what we do; being determined to improve, by adopting and sharing the best practice we can find; and making our own contribution more valuable through continuous personal development, comparing ourselves with the best; and by listening to the people we serve.'

And here is what it 'looks' like . . .

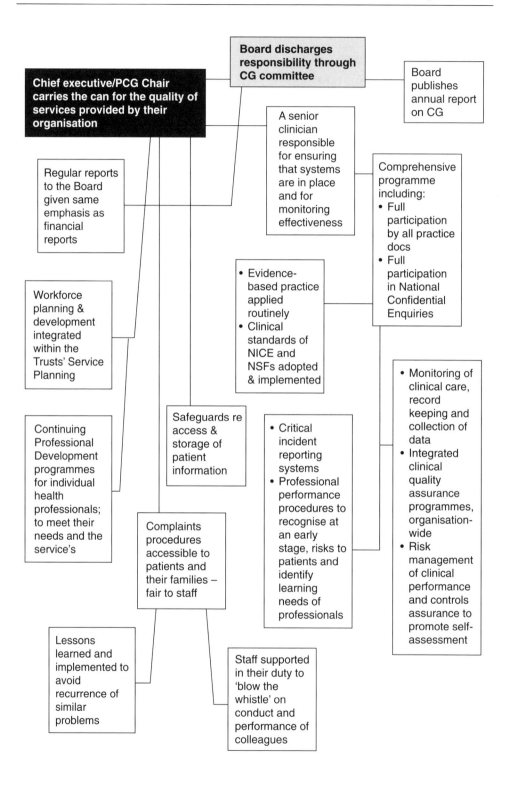

If you haven't got around to it yet, now is a good time to make a cup of coffee, delve into the archive of bumph from the DoH and read the White Paper *A First Class Service*.

If you want to cheat, here are the five headline issues.

In short the aim is to:

1 tackle the causes of ill-health
2 make services quick and easy to use
3 ensure the consistency of services – regardless of where you live
4 try and provide joined-up services that are not constrained by artificial barriers between services such as health and social services
5 spend money on equipment, building and staff.

Get the idea? Let's see . . .

😊 Exercise

Think about the aims in the five headings above and write down what part clinical governance could play in delivering them.

We are all going to get 10 years for this!

Relax, we are not going to jail! In the first White Paper, *The New NHS: Modern, Dependable*, they, whoever 'they' are, who wrote it, envisaged a 10-year programme of rolling improvement in the NHS.

Haven't read *Modern, Dependable* – shame on you! We'll let you cheat just one more time; it only said three main things about quality. Here they are:

1 Clear national standards, delivered through National Service Frameworks and the National Institute of Clinical Excellence.
2 Local delivery of quality services, delivered through CG and a statutory duty of quality (maybe you will end up in jail after all!), supported by lifelong learning programmes and professional self-regulation.
3 Monitoring of services through the Commission for Health Improvement (the NHS regulatory body we call *Off-sick*) and the NHS Performance

Framework. Oh, sorry, we nearly forgot; and the patient and user experience survey (expected to report that the doctors and the nurses were **luverley** . . .).

Joining all that together is the concept of CG. Or, in other words:

> 'A framework through which NHS organisations are accountable for continuously improving the quality of their services and safeguarding high standards of care by creating an environment in which excellence in clinical care will flourish.'

Let's take a closer look at some of the issues.

MOVE UP THE CURVE OR GO TO JAIL . . .

In the language of management guru-speak there is a phrase. It is 'the quality curve'. What it means is that at one end of the scale you will find organisations that work at the leading edge of quality and are world-class and at the other end, there are the poor performers. Generally we discover organisations, whether they are health organisations or not, around the middle of the curve.

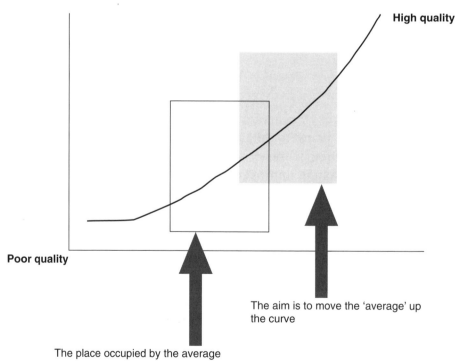

High quality

Poor quality

The aim is to move the 'average' up the curve

The place occupied by the average

Part of the NHS's response, to get more of its organisations to move up the quality curve, is to introduce a concept called 'the statutory duty' of quality.

In other words: move up the curve or go to jail.

> What difference will threatening people with sanctions and punishment make to real quality in the NHS? Will the thought of appearing in the dock, or being dragged before the Health Select Committee really make a district nurse, on her sixth visit of the day, in rainy, freezing cold, downtown Liverpool (sorry Liverpool) really make her do the job better? What does a statutory duty mean to you?

LEARNING FROM THE BEST

The question really worth asking is: who decides 'what's best'? You might want to think about that, too.

> Have a think . . . What really motivates people to do their jobs better? Threats, money, encouragement? What motivates you?

Anyway, there have been plenty of recent examples where anything but the best has emerged. The idea of CG is to cascade good practice into the NHS as fast as possible. In effect, learning from leading-edge outfits and getting them to pass on what they do.

What does that mean for you and your organisation?

The risk is that you could be blindly carrying on with a procedure that everyone else stopped doing ages ago. Perhaps prescribing less than optimally or even managing clinical governance in a cack-handed way.

There are three important things to remember about clinical governance:

- Appoint a good CG lead, someone with interest, enthusiasm and authority to act.
- Do whatever is necessary to keep up-to-date with best practice – the phrase you don't want to hear is: 'Well, well, I never knew that . . .'.
- Audit everything you do and compare it with what everyone else is doing.

. . . do that and sleep at night.

ANNEX – STOP PRESS!

Whilst this book was in preparation two events emerged which will have a long-term bearing on clinical practice, risk management and how practices are organised. They are far reaching and very significant.

But for the flexibility of modern book production we would not have been able to include them, so we are grateful to the publishers for allowing us the opportunity to add this last minute annex just days before going to press.

☢ THE FUTURE OF PROFESSIONAL REGULATION

Throughout the book we make reference to the General Medical Council. The GMC regulates the medical profession – but, perhaps, not for much longer.

Originally the GMC was set up to protect the profession from charlatans and poor practice. Over the years there has been a subtle shift.

At present the GMC, in its reform factsheet published in October 2004, says it has four main functions:

- keeping up-to-date registers of qualified doctors
- fostering good medical practice
- promoting high standards of medical education
- dealing firmly and fairly with doctors whose fitness to practise is in doubt.

. . . and the over-arching purpose, to protect, promote and maintain the health and safety of the community by ensuring proper standards in the practise of medicine.

The GMC has come in for some stinging criticism for being too doctor focused and too slow in responding to allegations of poor practice. GMC disciplinary hearings are not designed to allay public anxieties and they appear unable to reconcile the competing requirements of identifying poorly performing or negligent doctors and protecting patients. Full details of what they are up to can be ferreted out at www.gmc-uk.org. We do mean ferret, their website is comprehensive but complex, with tiny print and at the time of writing the link to the NHS complaints procedure was out of date and took you to the wrong site!

In brief they proposed a reduction in size of the ruling Council, a shift in the balance of membership, towards more lay members (who remained in a minority) and a sprucing-up of the license to practice and revalidation processes, which, in 2001, attracted a vote of no confidence from the BMA. They also attempted to streamline their complaints and disciplinary procedures.

For critics of the GMC – and they have plenty – the changes were too little and too late.

The crux of the problem is that the GMC is an organisation that is funded by the subscriptions of doctors. Just think for a moment. If you were obliged to subscribe to a club, I guess you'd want the rules to be in your favour. However, it struggles to claim it is independent and exists for patients, too.

The GMC was struggling on in a no-man's land of pleasing no-one and then came the bombshell in the guise of Dame Janet Smith.

Just in case you have been attempting a solo-round-the-world tunnelling record and are unaware of who Dame Janet is, she is the judge who has been conducting the public inquiry into the Harold Shipman affair. If you are not aware of who Shipman was, go and get a job on an Artic ice breaker. Shipman has turned out to be a GP, a drug addict, a convincing liar and Britain's most prolific mass murderer. Not surprisingly, Dame Janet and a few hundred relatives, patients, the public, the press and the rest of the world wanted to know how Shipman could have got away with his criminal activities for so long?

In the sixth volume of her report into Shipman, Dame Janet lit the fuse on the future of the GMC. This is how the BBC's excellent webnews service http://newswww.bbc.net.uk/1/hi/health/4081425.stm reported the events on the day of her announcement:

Shipman report demands GMC reform

Harold Shipman is believed to have killed at least 215 patients. **The General Medical Council is doing too little to protect patients, the latest report from the Shipman Inquiry has said.**

The report criticises the GMC for 'looking after its own' and recommends a radical shake-up in its structure.

The GMC says it is making wholesale changes, but the report said its reforms did not go far enough.

The inquiry was set up in 2001 after GP Harold Shipman's conviction in a bid to prevent such events occurring again.

Main recommendations:

- Change GMC structure to remove medical majority.
- The GMC to no longer have sole responsibility for assessing doctors' fitness to practise.
- The GMC to be directly accountable to Parliament.
- Improvements to the way doctors' performance is assessed.
- A central NHS database containing information on all doctors.
- Systems to be in place to allow staff to raise concerns.

Dame Janet said: 'I cannot guarantee that, if all my recommendations are implemented, it will be impossible for a doctor who is determined to kill a patient to do so without detection.

'But I believe that, if my recommendations are introduced, the deterrent effect will be considerable, and the chances of a doctor such as Shipman escaping detection will be very much reduced.'

In the report, Dame Janet accepted that the GMC had introduced changes to the way it works in light of the Shipman case.

'I have concluded there has not yet been the change of culture within the GMC that will ensure that patient protection is given the priority it deserves.'

Dame Janet said she believed the GMC should be given the opportunity to put its house in order.

But she said its role in both investigating and punishing doctors, its fitness to practise procedures, should be split up.

Doctors should instead be disciplined by an independent body.

She also called for this to be reviewed in three to four years, with the potential for fitness to practise to be taken away from the GMC altogether if it was found to be wanting.

Ouch!

Undoubtedly stunned by the news, the GMC President Sir Graham Catto, said: 'I am certainly not complacent. I have introduced the most radical reform programme for medical regulation, not just in this country, but in any country.'

The GMC added that the public was involved in every stage of the process and there would be even greater involvement in the future.

In a statement, the GMC said: 'We are making every effort to make our own procedures accessible, streamlined and transparent, but we have long called for a "single portal" that could be the confidential first port of call for people with concerns.'

Dame Janet also called for a central database to be established containing information about every doctor working in the UK which would be accessible to both patients and NHS bodies.

Fine words, but they are unlikely to cut much ice with a government hell-bent on modernising the NHS and introducing a patient-focused service.

It got worse for the GMC when Dame Janet criticised their plans for a new system of revalidation (currently being finalised), which will involve regularly checking doctors' competency to practise, because doctors would not face objective tests which would allow their fitness to practise to be properly evaluated.

Health Secretary John Reid weighed in and accepted that more work was needed to reform the GMC. He said 'Standards of behaviour must be high and action against those who fail to maintain those standards must be timely, firm and fair. Nothing should be higher than the protection of patients.'

WHAT DOES ALL THIS ADD UP TO?

This book is being researched and written in the shadow of a General Election in late Spring 2005. It is unlikely that the government will take any action before that time; they certainly won't want to stir up a row with the doctors just before an election. After? It is inconceivable that we will return to the halcyon days of medicine when GPs were left in peace to go about their business in an atmosphere of trust and respect. Too much has happened.

The smart money says the regulation of the medical profession will be handed to the Healthcare Commission, or an off-shoot of it. Medical education will be for the employers and perhaps a new Council for Continuing Professional Medical Education.

One thing is pretty certain, the GMC will be left with the rump job of keeping a list of registered practitioners. These days that just means a computer and a website and it is difficult to imagine the resources required would be much more than a man and a dog in an office above a chip shop in the suburbs. Quite unlike the glass tower the GMC currently occupies at 350 Euston Road, London, pictured proudly on their website.

This would have a huge impact on the cost of registration. Presently, registration with the GMC costs £390 and there is an annual renewal fee of £290. Provisional registration costs £200. It is hard to see, in an IT-enabled system, why a renewal should cost no more than a few pounds and a straightforward registration no more than a hundred.

. . . WHAT DOES ALL THIS MEAN FOR YOU?

☺

Where, in the text of this book, we use the GMC to frighten you, bully you and make you sit up and take notice, in the passing of not too much time, you might have to go through the book and cross out GMC and write in something, or body, else.

One thing is for sure, the new arrangements will not frighten you, bully you or make you sit up and take notice. They will terrify you, intimidate you and keep you awake at night! Suddenly all the good advice in this book is even more valuable! (*Editor – make a note for the publisher to double the price of the third edition!*) It's an ill wind that blows nobody any good!

THERE'S MORE . . . CHAPERONES AND WHO IS WATCHING THE WATCHERS?

As if the events and consequences of the Shipman episode were not enough for the medical profession to cope with, there is more. Events surrounding the conviction of Folkestone GP, Clifford Ayling, also have far reaching consequences.

Ayling received a four-year prison sentence in December 2000 after being convicted of 13 indecent assaults on female patients between 1991 and 1998. During his trial, many more victims came forward and it will probably never be known how many he abused in total. Ayling steadfastly denied all the allegations and continues to do so.

Prior to his conviction Ayling had been sacked by no less than four hospitals, although, astoundingly, no further action was taken at the time. So outrageous was his behaviour that his conviction led to an official inquiry and the publication of a White Paper (Cmd 6298) in September 2003, followed by an independent investigation into how the NHS had handled allegations of his misconduct.

At the time, Health Secretary John Reid said:

> 'It is completely unacceptable that these events were allowed to happen. No patient should be left in a position where those in charge of their care are able to abuse their trust and take advantage. My sympathies go to the patients involved in this case.'

☺

Very good . . . but what are the implications of the recommendations in the report? Wait for it, hold on to your chair. The report says:

Several cases in Scotland, similar to that of Ayling, including the inappropriate examination of men, have lead Scottish courts to hand out jail sentences of up to nine years.

> '. . . trained chaperones should be available to all patients who are having intimate examinations.'

Practitioners are currently advised (and we reinforce this in this book) to offer patients a chaperone if they are carrying out intimate examinations, such as of the breasts, genitalia or rectum.

The recommendation that practitioners should use trained chaperones during intimate examinations is being considered by ministers.

The report is adamant: ' . . . there is a need for all NHS trusts to set out clear policies on chaperones to end the current confusion over what their role is, when they should be present and who they should be.'

Under present arrangements a chaperone may be 'any person' agreed to by the patient and the chaperone need not be in the room or have sight of the examination. Being in 'ear-shot' is considered adequate.

The report is clear in its intentions. The present arrangement should go. It says: '. . . no family member or friend, or untrained NHS administrative staff member should be expected to act as a formal chaperone.' It goes on: '. . . all trusts should make their chaperone policy explicit to patients and ensure there is enough funding to implement it.'

It is understood that the Secretary of State for Health is minded to recommend that 'Qualified Health Care Professionals' should be present to judge whether an examination is being carried out appropriately.

What are the implications?

- Practice nurses who are already under extreme pressure are unlikely to be available.
- Could nursing auxiliaries carry out the job? Who would recruit, train and pay for them?
- Doctors who fail to have a nurse present during intimate examinations might leave themselves open to accusation, prosecution and litigation as well as a jail sentence.
- Is it likely that male doctors could refuse to perform intimate examinations on women?

Is the problem confined to women patients and male doctors? Can we predict there will be complaints made by male patients that examinations by male and female doctors have been inappropriate? Remember the case of the three Sterling University students? Allan Buchan, a doctor at Stirling University, was jailed for two and a half years for molesting three male students during routine medical examinations.

The problem with accusations being made against doctors is that there is very little verifiable evidence. Most cases rely on the accuser's word and the police going on a fishing expedition, trying to find further patients wishing to make a complaint, to add weight to their case.

The system is open to abuse by unscrupulous patients. And it has to be said, dodgy policemen. What happens when the Old Bill asks the question: 'We are investigating Dr Bloggs for inappropriate examinations. Do you feel that Dr Bloggs examined you correctly?'

How might a patient know what the answer to the question is? How easy is it to turn doubt into innuendo, innuendo into implication and implication into allegation?

Place 20 young women in a witness box against one elderly doctor in the dock and who do the jury believe? The dirty old man or the abused women? Where is the truth and how is it discovered?

Recent surveys have shown that, despite being aware of the risk of suffering allegations of inappropriate behaviour or worse, only a minority of male doctors and very few female doctors regularly use a chaperone. Experienced GPs say that the vast majority of patients themselves do not want the privacy of their consultations interrupted by chaperones. When they are about to undergo intimate examinations, most patients refuse the offer of a chaperone. Understandable, perhaps, if the chaperone is a receptionist sitting outside an open door. If the option were to be a qualified nurse, would opinions change?

To protect themselves against false accusations of performing examinations for sexual gratification, practitioners will have to provide evidence and that can only be video evidence of the consultation, preparation and examination. Where does that lead us to?

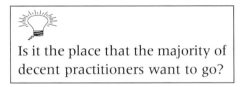

Is it the place that the majority of decent practitioners want to go?

Care to take a stab at calculating the resource implications for having qualified health professionals standing by on the off-chance a practitioner may need to perform an intimate examination? What are the implications for a single-handed practice?

Patients must be safe and have the right to be treated professionally. No right minded practitioner or manager would argue against it. However, what is the answer to the increasing welter of regulation, rules and guidance? We think the answer is TRUST. We have to be able to trust our practitioners, doctors, nurses and the managers who plan and run the services.

The question is: has the time for trust gone?

Have events such as Shipman and Ayling and others so eroded public and politicians' trust in the professions that external regulation is the only answer?

Has the GMC, slow and reluctant to criticise colleagues, so eroded public trust that self-regulation is no longer a viable option worth considering?

These are huge questions for the professions. It is also a huge challenge to the leadership of the professions – where are the leaders? We don't see any evidence of them stepping forward.

'I'm learning that trust and patience do not come naturally – they're like clothes, that I have to put on every morning.'
Gretchen Louise Glaser

'You may be deceived if you trust too much, but you will live in torment if you don't trust enough.'
Frank Crane

'Trust men and they will be true to you; treat them greatly and they will show themselves great.'
Ralph Waldo Emerson

'In God we trust – but keep your powder dry.'
Oliver Cromwell

INDEX

A First Class Service (DoH, 1998) 201
abbreviations in records 96
absences 183–4
access to buildings 151–2, 173–7
Access to Health Records Act (1990) 91–2
Access to Medical Reports Act (1988) 94
accident reporting and recording 155,
    168–70
    see also incident reporting and recording
active listening 49
anaesthesia 64–5
anti-virus software 139, 141
appendicitis 55
appointments
    missed 68
    patient expectations 116
    telephone skills 48, 117–18
appraisal processes 183
    and CPD 28
archive policies 141
audit
    and clinical governance 201–2, 204
    financial reporting measures 131–2
    and patient surveys 118–19
Australia, medical defence organisations 12

back safety 167, 186
back-ups 139
bad debts 118
balance sheets 124
battery and assault 76
body language 135
Bolam v *Friern Hospital Management
    Committee [1957]* 35–6, 42
Bolitho and others v *City and Hackney Health
    Authority [1997]* 36–7

bowel malignancies, clinical examinations
    53
brain tumours, clinical examinations 54
breach of contract 34–5
breast tumours, clinical examinations 54
building maintenance 151–2
    see also practice premises

cardiopulmonary resuscitation training 157
cash flow forecasts 124–5
causation 37, 41
chaperones 56, 107–9, 209–12
chemical disinfectants 161
chest pains 55
children
    competency and consent issues 80–2,
        86
    medication issues 58
CHRE *see* Council for Healthcare Regulatory
        Excellence
Civil Procedure Rules (1998) 39
claim forms 43
claims
    indemnity management 14
    negligence cases 36–8
    outcome and incidence data 45
    scope 9, 10–11
    see also legal processes
claims-made indemnity 10–11
cleaning fluids 161
clinical examinations 52–6
    appearances 52
    common pitfalls 53–6
    history-taking 53, 54, 55
    patient chaperones 56, 107–9
    physical examinations 54–6

214

prohibition notices 155–6
protective clothing 167
public liability insurance 148

quality considerations 197–8
  and clinical governance 201–3
questionnaires, patient surveys 118–19

radiation hazards 171–2
radio interviews 195
ramps 174, 177
reception areas 116–17
  access considerations 174–5, 176–7
  identifying risks 142–6
  privacy factors 85
record-keeping
  general principles 95–101
  see also medical records
recruitment issues 179–83
  contracts 182
  employee recommendations 180
  handbooks 182–3
  interviews 181–2
reflective practice, and CPD 26, 27
refusing treatment
  adults 78
  children 80–2
religious observance 187
removing patients 68, 70–1, 74
repeat prescriptions 59
Reporting of Injuries, Diseases and
    Dangerous Occurrences Regulations
    (RIDDOR) (1995) 168–9
reports *see* medical reports
resuscitation training 157
revalidation, role of GMC 21
risk management 4, 5–6, 196
  definitions 3
  key principles 5–6, 142–3
risks, types 4
run-offs 13

safety signs 170
Scotland, patient consent issues 82
self-regulation 20
  and role of CHRE 23–4

see also General Medical Council (GMC)
settlement terms
  pre-trial 41–2
  see also compensation
sexual issues
  and doctor–patient relationships 102–3
  inappropriate behaviours and advances
    69, 103–4
sharps disposal 162–3
Shipman, Harold 20, 57, 206–8
sick leave 183–4
sight problems, practice design
    considerations 176–7
signs and notices 147–8
  safety 170
skill *see* competency
small claims courts 43
software
  bespoke vs. Windows-based systems
    137–8
  safety considerations 166
  virus checkers 139, 141
special damages 38
special needs trust funds 38
special waste 162–3
staff issues 117–18
  communication and telephone skills 48,
    117–18
  confidentiality training 85
  contracts of employment 182
  disciplinary procedures 184
  employee handbooks 182–7
  grievance procedures 184–5
  health and safety checks 149–50, 153
  holidays and absences 183–4
  individual responsibilities 153–4
  locum cover 112–14
  PC protocols 139–41
  PC workstation safety checks 163–6
  training needs 85, 117–18
standard of proof 37
standards of practice 7–9
  and documentation 77
statements *see* medical reports; witness
    statements
statutory regulatory bodies 20, 23–4